"For anyone who's ever struggled with thoughts of suicide or who has a loved one who does, this workbook is a must-have. Kathryn Gordon is kind and practical in her approaches to managing suicidal thoughts, and in helping us find what we might have lost during the many years of struggle—hope."

—**Janina Scarlet, PhD**, award-winning author of *Superhero Therapy*

"This book is outstanding—compassionate, packed with practical exercises, and based on research, theory, and clinical practice. It can help readers to suffer less, to stay safe, and to want to live. *The Suicidal Thoughts Workbook* stands alone just fine as a self-help book, and it also will be a good complement to psychotherapy."

—**Stacey Freedenthal, PhD, LCSW,** psychotherapist, associate professor of social work at the University of Denver, and author of *Helping the Suicidal Person*

"I am tremendously grateful for the opportunity to endorse this helpful tool. Having survived suicide attempts, I can honestly say that I wish I had something like this that could have helped me better understand everything that I was dealing with on the inside. Kathryn Gordon, thank you for thinking about those of us who struggle every day with this invisible illness—we are forever grateful."

—**Kevin Berthia**, suicide survivor/advocate/speaker, and founder of the Kevin Berthia Foundation

"Suicidal thoughts and feelings can sometimes end in death. And even if people don't act on them, suicidal thoughts are incredibly painful in the moment. The good news is that for many people, using the skills in this book can help them to cope with suicidal thoughts and intensely painful emotions. Studies show that most people who use skills like the ones in this book can significantly reduce their suffering and help them build a life worth living. It is possible to recover, and this book is a good place to start."

—**April C. Foreman, PhD, LP,** executive board member of the American Association of Suicidology

"*The Suicidal Thoughts Workbook* is a true gem in a world where suicide vulnerability exists in the shadows of shame and fear. Kathryn Gordon brilliantly weaves her professional expertise as a therapist and researcher to deliver a comprehensive workbook that breaks down each layer of suicide complexity, from 'why suicidal thoughts occur' to specific strategies for developing personalized solutions. Most impressively, the workbook is genuinely empowering, offering hope to those who might otherwise feel hopeless."

—**Rheeda Walker, PhD**, professor of psychology at the University of Houston, and author of *The Unapologetic Guide to Black Mental Health*

The Suicidal Thoughts Workbook

CBT SKILLS *to* REDUCE EMOTIONAL PAIN, INCREASE HOPE, *and* PREVENT SUICIDE

KATHRYN HOPE GORDON, PhD

New Harbinger Publications, Inc.

Publisher's Note

This publication is designed to provide accurate and authoritative information in regard to the subject matter covered. It is sold with the understanding that the publisher is not engaged in rendering psychological, financial, legal, or other professional services. If expert assistance or counseling is needed, the services of a competent professional should be sought.

NEW HARBINGER PUBLICATIONS is a registered trademark of New Harbinger Publications, Inc.

Distributed in Canada by Raincoast Books

Copyright © 2021 by Kathryn Hope Gordon
New Harbinger Publications, Inc.
5674 Shattuck Avenue
Oakland, CA 94609
www.newharbinger.com

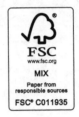 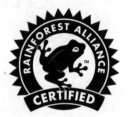

"Reasons for Living Inventory" adapted from Building a Life Worth Living: A Memoir, copyright © 2020 by Dr. Marsha M. Linehan. Used by permission of Random House, an imprint and division of Penguin Random House LLC.

Illustrations by Alyse Ruriani; Cover design by Amy Shoup; Acquired by Ryan Buresh; Edited by Jennifer Eastman

---

Library of Congress Cataloging-in-Publication Data

Names: Gordon, Kathryn H. (Kathryn Hope), author.
Title: The suicidal thoughts workbook / Kathryn Hope Gordon.
Description: Oakland, CA : New Harbinger Publications, Inc., [2021] | Includes bibliographical
   references.
Identifiers: LCCN 2020056683 | ISBN 9781684037025 (trade paperback)
Subjects: LCSH: Suicidal behavior--Prevention. | Suicidal behavior--Treatment.
Classification: LCC RC569 .G67 2021 | DDC 616.85/8445--dc23
LC record available at https://lccn.loc.gov/2020056683

Printed in the United States of America

23   22   21

10   9   8   7   6   5   4   3   2

To Keith, Lyla, Graham, Mom, Dad, Annie, and Linda, who have sparked so much love, joy, and meaning in my life.

To all who have struggled with suicidal thoughts, I hope you find comfort and help in these pages.

Contents

Worksheets and Exercises

Foreword

The US suicide rate has trended upward in recent years, and this was the case before 2020's travails. Of course, some of 2020's woes were unwelcome and unexpected—and others needed and overdue—but there is clear evidence that these experiences have stressed the American public. There is thus some likelihood that 2020 will be yet another year that sees more US suicide deaths than the previous year. Regardless of that, it is an established fact that from the early 2000s to 2018 (the latest year for which we have clear, official data), the US rate was on a steady and relentless climb—higher each year than the last, year after year. In this light, our technology in risk assessment, intervention, and prevention can be viewed as insufficient, or as if progress has stalled.

Yet the current book is hopeful. How can that be? For one thing, the book's author has a hopeful disposition, a fact to which I can attest, having known her for close to twenty years, and this hope animates the pages that follow. Her hopefulness is not hollow; it is hard-won through many years of clinical experience, and that is apparent in these pages as well.

Of course, it is possible to remain hopeful even when objective circumstances indicate pessimism. Are there objective reasons for optimism?

Yes. Preliminary 2019 data suggest a reversal in the upward climb of US suicide rates—a *decrease* in suicides from 2018. Moreover, the world's suicide rate is decreasing, a fact that is repeatedly overlooked by American authors. That the international rate was decreasing while the American rate was increasing suggests some American-centric drivers. There are a few candidates for such US-specific factors (e.g., the opiate crisis, our cultural relationship to violence). Another is how relatively hard it can be to disseminate and implement knowledge gains in a society as free and open as that of the United States, and also one with significant disparity.

Such factors make it quite possible for there to be real gains in suicide-related assessment and intervention *and* for there to be increasing suicide rates. Dr. Gordon's recommendations in this book represent real gains in assessment and treatment; the challenge is to disseminate and implement them widely and to diverse groups, and this hopeful and practical book launches that endeavor.

—Thomas Ellis Joiner Jr., PhD

CHAPTER 1

Introduction

Welcome!

I'm so glad you're looking for help with your suicidal thoughts. Please take a moment to recognize the strength you're showing by beginning this workbook. It takes courage to try something new when you're at a low point. I admire your willingness to do that, and I hope that you feel a sense of pride about working on your mental health. Your life is valuable, even if it doesn't feel that way right now. You won't have to do this alone. I'll walk you through each step and give you tips on finding others who can support you along the way. Throughout this workbook, I'll be here to remind you of your worth and to help you build a life that you want to live—one with less pain, more joy, and more meaning.

A Note for Concerned Friends and Family

This workbook was designed for adults who struggle with suicidal thoughts. If you're reading it because you're concerned about someone else, thank you for your loving action. I hope it's a useful guide as you seek to understand and help them. Your support may be a spark of light for people in their darkest times. I created appendix A to answer some of the questions that you may have on your mind.

A Note to Clinicians

If you're reading this workbook because you're a clinician who wants to help your patients, thank you for your dedication to providing the highest level of care. As clinicians, we are honored to be in spaces where people share their most vulnerable moments with us. Our patients' trust in us must be met with sensitive, ethical, and compassionate care. I hope that you find this workbook useful in your practice. I have included a list of additional resources in appendix B.

A Note to the Reader

If you're reading this workbook for yourself, consider sharing appendices A and B with people in your support network. It may lighten the load of educating others while you devote your energy to healing.

Who Am I?

As a therapist, I have worked with hundreds of patients who have struggled with suicidal thoughts and behaviors. Together, we have created personalized, effective treatment plans to make positive changes in their lives. As a scientist, I have closely read and contributed to the research literature that guided the exercises in this workbook. Crucially, I have also listened to the wisdom and stories of people who have lived through suicidal crises. Through this workbook, I'm sharing what I have learned so that you can apply that knowledge to your life.

I wrote this workbook because I want to empower you. I want you to trust yourself to skillfully cope with suicidal thoughts. Your life and your feelings are valuable, which is why each section of this workbook prioritizes self-compassion at a time when you need it the most. Let's work together to find ways for you to hurt less by (1) making changes in areas you can control, and (2) soothing suffering in the face of the hardships you can't control.

Why Do You Have Suicidal Thoughts?

People reach this point through many different paths, but all tend to have one thing in common: overwhelming emotional pain that makes death seem like the only escape. I want you to know that suicidal thoughts are not a sign that you're weak or flawed—or that you should feel ashamed. They are signs that you're in pain. It is understandable that you want relief from pain when it feels unbearable. That is why this workbook shares ways to reduce pain rather than telling you that you're wrong for wanting to escape it.

In addition to your personal circumstances, societal conditions make it hard for many people to get their emotional and physical needs met. Discrimination and unequal access to quality health care, education, housing, childcare, and other basic needs create stress and harm mental health (e.g., Li et al., 2011; Oh et al., 2019). As the theologian and human rights activist Desmond Tutu put it, "There comes a point where we need to stop just pulling people out of the river. We need to go upstream and find out why they're falling in." As mental health advocates fight for necessary upstream changes that address inequality, this workbook is here to provide you with tools when you feel like you're sinking.

If you've ever had a hard time finding or affording a therapist, please know that it's not your fault and that you're not alone. Many people struggle to find help in the current system and feel stuck. How did you receive this workbook? Was it through a therapist, or did you find it on your own through a bookstore, library, or website? However this book got into your hands, I'm glad you were able to access it. A major purpose of this book is to make therapy tools widely available to all who need them.

What to Expect

This workbook takes you through a process that is similar to therapy. It begins by asking you questions to increase awareness about the situations that prompt your suicidal thoughts and behaviors. Then the important work of making positive changes begins. I want to acknowledge that many of the aspects of your life that led to suicidal thoughts may have not been in your control. This workbook makes suggestions for you, but that does not mean that it is your fault. Rather, it is acknowledging how hard life can be and that having support and coping tools can help.

The Three-Step Theory of Suicide

The workbook is structured around the three-step theory of suicide (3ST; Klonsky and May, 2015), which builds on research and other leading theories of suicide (e.g., the interpersonal theory of suicide; Joiner, 2005). The 3ST helps uncover causes of suicidal thoughts and points to areas where changes can prevent suicide. There are sections on each part of the 3ST (pain and hope, connections, and the capability to attempt suicide).

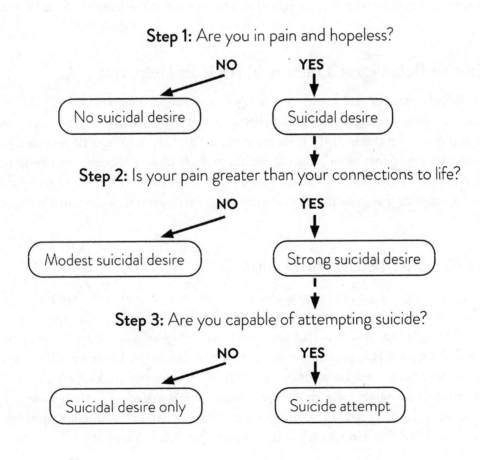

Figure adapted with permission from Klonsky et al., 2016

Overview of the Workbook

Chapter 2 will help you understand your suicidal thoughts and behaviors with a key message: you are not alone in your struggles. Next, chapter 3 describes the 3ST in more detail, so you can apply it to your life and explore the causes of your suicidal thoughts. Chapter 4 focuses on making a plan to cope with suicidal urges while staying safe. After you create a crisis plan, chapters 5 through 9 have in-depth exercises to provide relief from the hurt that drives suicidal thoughts. Chapter 5 focuses on problem solving and cognitive behavioral therapy (CBT) to reduce your emotional pain, while chapter 6 guides you through soothing suffering with self-compassion and acceptance. In chapter 7, we'll work together to increase hope with four strategies (seeking help, finding reasons for optimism, changing perspective, and attending to your emotions). You'll learn how to strengthen relationships in chapter 8 and to increase meaning in chapter 9. Then, chapter 10 provides guidance for creating and maintaining physical and emotional safety. The workbook concludes with chapter 11, which reviews what you've learned and helps you plan for the future.

How Cognitive Behavioral Therapy Skills Can Help You

Many of the workbook exercises were inspired by CBT, a type of science-supported therapy that is used to treat depression, eating disorders, insomnia, anxiety, suicidal thoughts, and other types of mental health problems (Beck, 1993; Linehan, 1993; Tarrier et al., 2008). CBT helps you (1) become aware of the thoughts and behaviors that worsen mental health, and (2) change thoughts and behaviors to improve mental health. In addition to CBT strategies, this workbook will focus on relationship- and emotion-based coping skills that make it easier to approach yourself and your feelings in a kind, helpful manner.

Basics of Cognitive Behavioral Therapy

When you're suffering, it's hard to imagine seeing your life in a different way. Hearing people say "look on the bright side" or "every cloud has a silver lining" can feel dismissive or can lead to shame for not being able to do so. It's not your fault that your mind seems stuck in a certain spot. Your pain and feelings are real and not something you can just snap out of by trying to think positive. CBT guides you through a step-by-step process toward new perspectives that ring true for you. Beck (1979) identified four common types of beliefs among people with suicidal thoughts: *Life is pointless, Life is miserable and must be escaped, I'm a burden on others,* and *I cannot cope with my problems.* Do you relate to any of those? This workbook includes chapters that address each of those beliefs, but first, let's look at a CBT model:

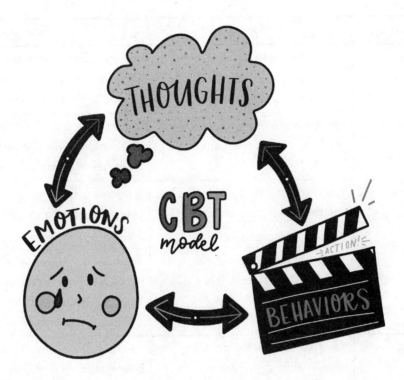

Illustration by Alyse Ruriani

CBT proposes that your thoughts, emotions, and behaviors all influence each other. What are you thinking about this workbook right now? If you think it will be helpful, you might feel excited or hopeful. If you think that it might work for other people, but not you, you probably feel down. If you're approaching it with an open mind, you likely feel curious. Your emotions also affect your thoughts and behaviors. If you feel irritable, you are more likely to think people are annoying, so you behave in irritated ways (e.g., snapping at people). Similarly, your behaviors and actions impact your thoughts and emotions. For example, if you make a mistake at work, you will be more likely to have negative thoughts (e.g., *I shouldn't have messed that up*) and painful emotions (e.g., embarrassment).

Thinking Patterns

Now that you understand ways that thoughts can influence feelings and behavior, let's look at some common thinking errors that lead to painful emotions (also called "cognitive distortions") developed by Beck (1979), Burns (1980), Ellis (2016), and others.

Thinking Error	Description	Example
All-or-nothing thinking	You view something in extremes (black and white) instead of in-between (gray areas).	You planned to exercise three days per week, but you missed a day. You decide the week was a fitness failure.
Overgeneralization	You think one negative experience applies to all similar situations.	You go on a date that doesn't go well. You decide you're doomed to have bad dates from now on.
Discounting the positive	You dismiss evidence that contradicts your negative views.	Someone compliments you. You tell yourself that they are just being nice and don't mean it.
Mind reading	You assume someone else's intent or the way they feel without evidence.	You texted someone, but it's been two hours, and they haven't responded. You assume it means they're mad or don't care about you.
Fortune telling	You assume something bad will happen without evidence.	You have an upcoming social event and believe that it will go poorly.
Emotional reasoning	You *feel* something is true and believe it to be true despite contrary evidence.	You ask a friend for a favor. They say they're happy to help, but you feel like a burden for asking. You conclude that you *are* a burden.
Shoulding	You tell yourself that you, others, or situations are supposed to be different.	You're upset that you and a friend grew apart and tell yourself, "I shouldn't be so sad. I should be over this by now."
Labeling	You take individual behaviors and interpret them as having a global meaning about you or others.	You are impatient with your child after a long day. You tell yourself that you're a bad parent.
Personalization	You think that something that is not about you is about you.	Your partner is in a bad mood (because of an experience they had at work), but you think it must be because you did something wrong.
Catastrophizing	Something bad happens, and your mind jumps to the worst-case scenario.	You feel embarrassed about something you said to a neighbor. You think they'll end your friendship and tell all the other neighbors to stop talking to you.

Which thinking errors do you relate to the most? Can you think of recent times where you've experienced some of them? We all experience them from time to time. It's part of being human. You're not doing this on purpose, and you're not to blame for having them. In fact, Beck (1979) called these types of thoughts "automatic." The good news is that once you can identify them, you can respond when your mind is telling you things that are not true. We'll return to CBT in more detail later. For now, let's talk about how to get the most from this workbook.

How to Use This Workbook

I recommend reading the workbook from beginning to end—rather than skipping around—to get the full impact of the material. The sequence was designed with intention and based on my experiences conducting therapy with people with suicidal thoughts. I have included a variety of exercises to meet the needs of the diverse individuals reading this book. I suggest that you try each exercise at least a few times. After you have tried them all, you may want to focus on the ones that you find most helpful in your life. It's best to have multiple go-to coping strategies rather than just one or two, because some may become ineffective when used over and over. A common mistake that I see in therapy is that people try a strategy once, decide it doesn't work, and then give up. It's totally understandable to feel that way when you don't see immediate benefits from the tool you used. However, taking care of your mental health is actually a lot like taking care of your physical health. If you start eating more nutritious foods, getting more sleep, and exercising more, you tend to see the strongest effects over time, with repeated healthy behaviors, rather than just after a few days or tries.

You can work through this workbook on your own, with a therapist, or with someone else you trust. People have different levels of access to mental health services, depending on finances, community availability, and other circumstances. As mentioned earlier, a major motivation for creating this workbook was to provide information to people who run into obstacles while seeking therapy. Nonetheless, know that it is often more challenging for people to work through these issues without the help of a therapist. Therefore, you may want to ask for support when you get stuck.

Prepare for Change

Now that you know what to expect from the workbook, let's focus on preparing for change. When you're at a low point in your life, the prospect of working through hardships can feel overwhelming. That is why I usually start therapy by asking people to identify their reasons for wanting to change (Miller and Rollnick, 2013; Britton et al., 2011). How much do you want change right now? Why do you want to change? Let's explore this in the worksheet below. After you fill it out, you can return to it whenever you need to remind yourself why you're doing the hard work of improving your mental health.

In the exercise below, select your reasons for wanting change, and feel free to add your own. Later, you can look at this list again when your desire for change starts slipping. Some people find it helpful to put their list in a prominent place (e.g., the refrigerator, a bedroom wall, a bathroom mirror) or take a picture of it with their phone so that it's easily accessed in moments of need. (A copy of this list is available on the New Harbinger website for downloading and printing: http://www.newharbinger.com /47025.)

Why I Want Change

- ☐ I want to feel better.
- ☐ I want life to hurt less.
- ☐ I want to be more present with my loved ones.
- ☐ I want to learn to cope with suicidal thoughts in healthier ways.
- ☐ I want more tools for experiencing and expressing my emotions.
- ☐ I want to learn new strategies for dealing with stressors.
- ☐ I don't want to feel helpless.
- ☐ I want to feel more control in my life.
- ☐ I want to feel hopeful.
- ☐ I want a more meaningful life.
- ☐ I want to enjoy life more.
- ☐ I want to be kinder to myself.
- ☒ I want to get better at accepting myself.
- ☐ I want to feel more comfortable with my emotions.
- ☐ I want to be there for my children (or partner, friends, or family).
- ☐ I want to feel safe.
- ☒ I want to be more authentic with others.
- ☐ I don't want my mental health struggles to hold me back from reaching my goals.
- ☐ _____
- ☐ _____
- ☐ _____

When people lack confidence, their motivation for change may dip. How confident do you feel about your ability to change? The exercise below includes a list of statements designed to boost your belief in yourself and your ability to change.

Confidence Boosters

Put a check mark next to all of the statements that apply, and feel free to add your own. If you're having a hard time coming up with examples, you can ask a therapist or loved one to help with this section. You can also try thinking about yourself as a friend: If you were your friend, what positive qualities would you see? You can return to this list whenever your confidence starts to drop.

- ☒ I'm kind.
- ☐ I'm thoughtful.
- ☐ I'm funny.
- ☐ I'm creative.
- ☐ I'm good at problem solving.
- ☒ I'm compassionate.
- ☐ I'm spiritual.
- ☐ I'm insightful.
- ☐ I'm a hard worker.
- ☒ I'm a good listener.
- ☒ I'm trustworthy.
- ☐ I'm brave.
- ☐ I'm patient.
- ☒ I'm appreciative.
- ☐ I'm fun to be around.
- ☒ I treat people fairly.
- ☒ I'm generous.
- ☐ I can take small steps to make my life better. I don't have to change everything at once.
- ☐ Other people who experiencing suicidal thoughts have been able to make changes even though they felt they couldn't. If they can do it, I can too.
- ☐ When I feel overwhelmed or backslide, that is okay and a normal part of the process. I can try again.

☐   I have made it through hard times before. List at least one example:

_____

☐   I have people who can help me through this. List at least one example:

_____mom & sister_____

☐   I have made changes before. List at least one example:

_____

☐   I have positive qualities that will help me through this. List at least one example:

_____

☐   I am capable of learning new skills. List at least one example:

_____

When Should I Seek Professional Help?

Most people with suicidal thoughts do not act on them. The thoughts, on their own, do not mean that you are at high risk of a suicide attempt. However, it's useful to recognize signs that your thoughts have become dangerous and might drive you to suicide (Chu et al., 2015). If it's hard to seek help when you're in a high-risk state, sharing a list of warning signs with loved ones can help (see the list below and appendix A). This can prompt them to offer extra support when they notice the signs and to make special efforts to check in with you at those times. That relieves some of the pressure on you to identify warning signs and find help all on your own.

If you are currently experiencing one or more of the warning signs listed below, please reach out for help right away. You can contact a crisis hotline, a mobile mental health service, a therapist, a medical professional, or other types of emergency care for help. You can also look within your support network to see if there are friends or relatives who will stay with you until the crisis has passed or who will accompany you to the emergency room if you decide you would like to go there. You are worthy of help. You are loved, and you belong. I want you to be safe and get the support you need to hold on.

Warning Signs

- specific plans for how or when you will kill yourself

- intent to act on plans to kill yourself

- getting (or plans to get) something to kill yourself with (e.g., a gun, drugs to overdose on)

- high levels of agitation

- significant increase in sleep disturbances (e.g., nightmares, insomnia)

- significant weight loss without an intention to lose weight

- isolating yourself from others

- withdrawing from relationships

- the feeling that you cannot control your urges to kill yourself

- neglect of basic self-care, hygiene, and safety (e.g., eating, bathing, brushing your teeth, taking prescribed medications for medical conditions)

Thank You

When you're in a dark place and want to end your life, it is one of the toughest yet most necessary moments to care for your mental health needs. Change is hard, and it takes time. Please be patient with yourself. From the bottom of my heart, I want to thank you for hanging in there with me. You are valuable. Your life matters, and I want to help you navigate it with the wisdom of science, clinical practice, and the stories of people who have faced their own suicidal crises.

Summary of Key Points

- Suicidal thoughts are driven by emotional pain. They are not your fault. Suicidal thoughts do not mean that you are a weak or flawed person.

- This workbook will use the 3ST framework and CBT techniques to help you effectively cope with your suicidal thoughts.

- You should seek additional help right away if you're experiencing the warning signs listed above.

Reflection

What thoughts, ideas, and feelings did you have while reading and working through this chapter? Were there certain parts you didn't relate to? What parts did you relate to most? What did you learn? I recommend keeping a journal as you read through the workbook, so that you can write down ideas that you want to remember, process your thoughts, and express your emotions along the way.

CHAPTER 2

Understand Your Suicidal Thoughts

Now that you have an overview of the workbook, let's focus on better understanding your suicidal thoughts and how they are affected by your environment. I'll begin by describing different kinds of suicidal thoughts and behaviors and how commonly they occur. Then we'll take time to reflect on your personal story. Too often when people hear that someone is suicidal, they jump to urging them to seek safety before asking about the pathway that brought them there. Even if they mean well, it can still feel bad. Has that ever happened to you? If it has, I'm sorry that you experienced that. Your journey is important, and we'll take time to explore it together in this chapter.

Understanding your suicidal thoughts will help you effectively apply the workbook exercises to your life. As we explore them, I want to note that suicidal thoughts can happen following a specific stressful event or a combination of factors. Other times, suicidal thoughts feel like they are coming out of nowhere. Having difficulty pinpointing the source of distress can cause anxiety or frustration. If that is the case for you, know that it is okay. Please just write whatever comes to your mind, and that will be useful. You can always revisit the exercises later if you have new insights.

If you prefer to use art (e.g., drawing, painting, a collage) or some other type of creative method to express yourself in these exercises besides writing, feel free to do that. Sometimes people feel most free expressing their emotions through art instead of words. There is no wrong way to do this. I appreciate you giving it a try. I know you can do it!

Types of Suicidal Thoughts and Behaviors

There are three types of suicidal thoughts and behaviors I'll discuss in this section: suicidal ideation, nonsuicidal self-injury, and suicide attempts.

Suicidal ideation (referred to as "suicidal thoughts" throughout this workbook) is having thoughts about ending your life with some desire for death. Suicidal thoughts can be experienced in many different ways. Some people have frequent suicidal thoughts (e.g., daily, multiple times per day) while others experience them less often (e.g., once every few years, only in times of intense distress). Suicidal thoughts also range from fleeting thoughts that last seconds or minutes to more intense, persistent thoughts that last hours, days, or longer.

Therapists often note the difference between passive suicidal thoughts (e.g., *If I were in a life-threatening situation, I wouldn't go out of my way to survive* or *I wouldn't mind getting into a bad car accident or falling asleep and never waking up*) and active ones (e.g., *I'll kill myself when I get a chance* or *I want to end my life*). Passive suicidal thoughts tend to reflect a desire to die without intent or plans to kill yourself, while active suicidal thoughts involve some level of planning or intent to kill yourself.

Passive suicidal thoughts can persist for long periods of time, never becoming active suicidal thoughts. Suicidal thoughts can also switch between passive and active depending on distress levels and situational circumstances. There are people who experience suicidal thoughts in all kinds of different ways. How frequent are your suicidal thoughts? Do they tend to be passive, active, or both? Have you noticed certain patterns for when they tend to emerge (e.g., high stress times, following sleep deprivation, during certain parts of the menstrual cycle; Owens and Eisenlohr-Moul, 2018)? Reflecting on those patterns, perhaps in your journal, can help you better understand yourself and times of vulnerability.

Sometimes images, urges, or thoughts of suicide flash into people's minds even though they don't want to die. In one study, 431 college students were asked if they ever imagined jumping when in a high place. Around half of the respondents reported that they had imagined it at least once in their lives (Hames et al., 2012). While the experience was more common among people who had considered suicide at some point in their lives (74 percent) than those who hadn't (43 percent), people who never considered suicide said they imagined jumping from a high place too. Why do these thoughts pop into our minds? Scientists are unsure, but some think that our brains are trying to warn us to step back and stay safe (Hames et al., 2012).

For most people who are not suicidal, these thoughts pop into their minds and then pop right back out. However, some people with obsessive-compulsive disorder (OCD) continue to have more persistent, unwanted thoughts of self-harm (e.g., an image of driving into oncoming traffic). These are called "intrusive thoughts" or "obsessions." They cause distress for the person having them and often lead to repetitive behaviors (compulsions) to reduce the distress (e.g., avoiding knives, pills, high places, or driving). This workbook does not focus on these types of thoughts. If you're having those experiences, please see appendix B for a workbook suggestion specifically for overcoming OCD with thoughts of self-harm (Hershfield, 2018) and seek professional help. There are effective treatments available.

Nonsuicidal self-injury (NSSI) is intentionally damaging one's body tissue (e.g., by cutting or burning) without any intent to die as a result. Because people with NSSI commonly experience suicidal thoughts, we will explore this a bit. However, it's important to seek more comprehensive care for NSSI through a therapist or a workbook specifically designed for it (see appendix B for information about Gratz and Chapman, 2009).

Suicide attempts include nonfatal potentially self-injurious acts with some intent to die as a result. The term is purposely broad so that it includes suicide attempts that range between less and more medically dangerous and low and high levels of intent to die.

Now that you understand these different types of suicidal thoughts and behaviors, let's reflect on your personal experiences.

My Story

This worksheet will ask what situation prompted the thought or behavior and how you coped with it. If it's hard to pinpoint something precisely, that is okay. You can write that you're not sure in those spaces. I encourage you to be gentle with yourself as you process your feelings and past experiences.

1. How old were you when you first had a suicidal thought? _____

    What prompted the thought?

    _____

    _____

    _____

    _____

    _____

    _____

    _____

2. How old were you when you had your most recent suicidal thought? _____

    What prompted the thought?

    _____

    _____

    _____

    _____

    _____

    _____

    _____

3. How have you coped with suicidal thoughts in the past?

    _____

    _____

    _____

    _____

4. Have you attempted suicide? (circle one):   **no   yes, once   yes, multiple times**

    If yes, how old were you at the time(s) and what prompted the suicide attempt(s)?

    _____

    _____

    _____

    _____

    What happened after the suicide attempt?

    _____

    _____

    _____

    _____

    How did you feel afterward? How do you feel about it now?

    _____

    _____

    _____

    _____

Feelings About Suicidal Thoughts

Sometimes judgmental reactions to suicidal thoughts come from your own mind and lead to shame and avoidance that interfere with your ability to work through them. Let's spend some time identifying your reactions so that you can recognize and counter shame while completing this workbook. Consider the situations below:

Sonia was laid off from her job and struggled to find new work. She lost her health insurance and was unable to find a therapist she could afford for three months. Her mother told her that she could move back home, but she felt embarrassed about doing that in her thirties. For the first time in her life, Sonia started thinking about killing herself. She was scared that it meant she was "going crazy." Sonia told herself a lot of people had it worse than her and that she should be more grateful. These thoughts led to feeling more out-of-control and guilty.

Carl grew up feeling trapped in an emotionally abusive home. He learned at an early age that he felt less trapped when considering suicide. Even though he never acted on it and never intended to, he often found himself going back to imagining his death during stressful times. He felt comforted and ashamed at the same time. He told a friend about his suicidal thoughts. The friend was shocked, and Carl realized he had become so used to suicidal thoughts that he felt numb.

Next, we'll process your reactions to your suicidal thoughts and behaviors. People experience a range of thoughts and emotions in response to their suicidal thoughts. No matter what your feelings are, it's okay to have them.

My Reactions to My Suicidal Thoughts

Throughout this exercise, examples have been provided to guide you.

Thought: Other people can handle stress just fine. I must be broken.

How did that make you feel?

Ashamed. I should be able to deal with stress without falling apart. Other people have harder lives and they handle things just fine. I must be lazy or weak or just damaged. I didn't want anyone to know I was thinking about suicide. Whenever someone asked how I felt, I always said "good" or "fine." I wish just one of them would have seen how I really felt inside. I wanted to hide, but I also wanted someone to help me. It was a painful mix of feelings.

Thought: _____

_____

How did that make you feel?

_____

_____

_____

_____

_____

Thought: _____

_____

How did that make you feel?

_____

_____

_____

_____

_____

Thought: _____

_____

How did that make you feel?

_____

_____

_____

_____

_____

Other People's Reactions to My Suicidal Thoughts

Your reactions to your suicidal thoughts may be influenced by other people's responses. Hopefully, you have had positive experiences where people reacted with support, love, and kindness. Some people are wonderful at figuring out how to help people who are hurting. Others may jump to problem solving, dismiss your pain, or contact emergency services without first trying to understand your perspective.

Let's consider your experiences with others. First, we'll start with Logan's story, followed by Logan's worksheet as an example.

Logan has bipolar disorder and had a manic episode that led to involuntary hospitalization. Once he got out of the hospital, he told himself he would stay on his medication, go to therapy, and make sure he never ended up in the hospital again. Logan started off feeling well but then began to feel drained by the pressure from his family to prove that he was happy and functioning well. He found his mind drifting into fantasies about suicide to relieve the strain. Afterward, Logan felt ashamed for thinking about suicide as an option. He thought it made him sinful for not trusting God to bring him out of it, as he had learned growing up.

Other People's Reactions to My Suicidal Thoughts (Logan's Example)

Person: My grandfather

Response: "If your faith in God was strong enough, you wouldn't think those dark thoughts anymore. You have to trust in Jesus and just pray. I don't even know why you need those medications. I don't take any when I'm going through hard times."

How did that you feel about that? I regretted telling my grandfather. Part of my recovery plan in the hospital was that I would share my feelings with my family. On the one hand, I feel like he just doesn't really understand mental illness. He's from a different generation and doesn't know better. But another part of me feels horrible for letting him down. I don't want him to worry about me or think I'm not strong enough in my faith.

Person: My sister

Response: "I know we weren't supposed to talk about our feelings growing up, but I have had those thoughts sometimes too. I think it runs in our family. Grandma might have had bipolar disorder or something like it. They just didn't know much about it then and called her 'crazy' instead."

How did you feel about that? Talking to my sister helped me feel less alone. I have so much respect for my sister. Hearing that she also had suicidal thoughts made it clear to me that this wasn't something that just happens to bad or weak people. She's one of the strongest people I know. I thought what she said about my grandma was interesting. It made me sad to think there's still misunderstanding about how having bipolar disorder affects people and what's out of their control. I guess it made me feel validated that my struggles were real and a little bit sad for myself that I felt pressure to put on a happy face.

Now fill in the worksheet with your own experiences.

Other People's Reactions to My Suicidal Thoughts

Person: _____

Response: _____

_____

_____

_____

How did you feel about that?

_____

_____

_____

_____

Person: _____

Response: _____

_____

_____

_____

How did you feel about that?

_____

_____

_____

_____

I hope you feel accomplished after processing your past experiences with suicidal thoughts and behaviors. In the next section, I'll show you that whatever your past experiences have been like, you are not alone in your struggles, and you are not to blame for your suicidal thoughts. We will also explore how cultural and other factors are related to suicide. Then I'll shift from generalizations and statistics to asking how these factors have specifically influenced you. Developing these insights will help you respond to your suicidal thoughts with awareness and acceptance instead of confusion and self-criticism.

How Common Are Suicidal Thoughts and Behaviors?

Worldwide, we lose approximately eight hundred thousand people to suicide every year (World Health Organization, 2019). Suicide was the tenth leading cause of death among US adults in 2018, with approximately 48,344 people tragically dying this way—14.8 out of every 100,000 people (Drapeau and McIntosh, 2020). Beyond that, there were far more suicide attempts. Researchers believe that there are twenty to thirty suicide attempts for every suicide death (Han et al., 2016). While most people who attempt suicide do not go on to die by suicide, many continue to struggle with the thoughts (Owens et al., 2002). These statistics mean that a lot of people are hurting and that many of us have lost loved ones to suicide. Approximately half of all people in the United States know someone who died by suicide (Cerel et al., 2018), and many find themselves in a deep state of grief as a result.

If suicide affects so many people, how can your experiences make you feel so alone? In recent years, more people (including celebrities) have publicly shared their struggles with suicidal thoughts. Social media has made it easier than ever for people to connect about their mental health experiences. Increased public understanding appears to have decreased stigma and led to more open discussions than there used to be (e.g., Smith et al., 2010). Still, some prejudice about suicide persists. Some people incorrectly think that suicidal thoughts are markers of flaws (e.g., being weak; Sand et al., 2013). This might lead you to think that you're blameworthy for having suicidal thoughts. This may have led you to hide that you have thoughts about killing yourself. Please know that others are doing the same. That means that you don't really know how many people in your life have struggled. I guarantee that people you know have also struggled with their mental health, even if you don't know about it. You're not alone in your experiences, and there are reasons to be hopeful for a future where more people can share their struggles without fear of judgment.

Who Is Affected by Suicidal Thoughts and Behaviors?

The Role of Mental Health

While most people with mental illnesses do not attempt suicide, Nock and colleagues (2009) found that approximately 80 percent of people in the United States who attempted suicide had a history of mental illness prior to their attempt. A more recent study by the Centers for Disease Control and Prevention (CDC) reported that 54 percent of people in the United States who died by suicide had no known mental illness (Stone et al., 2018). The CDC also reported that people who died by suicide—with or without a known mental illness—were likely to have experienced stressors or crises prior to their death (e.g., relationship problems, legal problems, eviction). While mental illnesses are associated with a higher likelihood of suicidal thoughts and behaviors, they are not typically strong predictors of suicide (Franklin et al., 2017) unless they're considered in combination with other factors (e.g., loneliness; Stickley and Koyanagi, 2016).

Researchers have found a higher suicide risk among people with substance-use problems, anorexia nervosa, depression, borderline personality disorder, and bipolar disorder (Chesney et al., 2014). There is also a link between opioid misuse and suicidal thoughts and behavior (Ashrafioun et al., 2017), and some have argued that some suicides are mistaken for unintentional opioid overdoses (Oquendo and Volkow, 2018). More comprehensive exploration is needed to fully understand suicide, because mental illness on its own is not a complete explanation. We'll explore how mental illness, along with other parts of your life, may be related to your suicidal thoughts in the next chapter. Please see appendix B for additional resources geared toward specific mental illnesses and seek professional help if you are affected by a mental illness and have not already received treatment.

The Role of Environments

In my own practice, I have worked with therapy patients with mental health issues that were worsened by a variety of environmental and societal conditions. I have worked with men who were taught that emotional expression meant weakness and with women whose pain was dismissed as overreacting. I have also worked with people who were rejected by their families for being gay or transgender and with immigrants who experienced discrimination while adjusting to a new country. Our families, communities, and broader culture influence our sense of self-worth, our coping responses, and our access to resources in times of need. These environmental factors may be part of the story of the group differences in suicide risk, which I'll explain in more detail below. First, let's reflect on your personal experiences.

Environmental Influences on My Mental Health

How was mental health viewed in the communities in which you grew up? Was it something that you could speak about openly?

_____

_____

_____

_____

Were medications and therapy viewed as appropriate ways to address mental health problems? How did this affect you?

_____

_____

_____

_____

How were emotions and seeking help viewed in the communities in which you grew up? Were you encouraged to be open or to keep your feelings private? When you asked for help, did you feel supported or dismissed?

_____

_____

_____

_____

How do you feel that culture at broader levels (e.g., the city, state, or country you live in currently or used to live in) has influenced your mental health?

_____

_____

_____

_____

What kinds of external circumstances do you think contribute to your pain and suicidal thoughts?

_____

_____

_____

_____

I hope that you found that exploration useful for understanding yourself and how your environment influences you. You're doing a great job thinking about these topics, which can be challenging to do. Before going into more statistics, I'll make two notes: (1) these are estimates (gathering accurate suicide data is complicated), and (2) any person, regardless of background or identity, can be affected by suicidal thoughts and behaviors. Within the United States, men are much more likely to die by suicide than women (23.4 versus 6.4 out of every 100,000) while women are much more likely to attempt suicide than men (about three times more likely; Drapeau and McIntosh, 2020). This pattern of higher suicide rates for men holds across most countries, though the specific numbers and proportions differ.

Suicide rates also seem to differ by ethnic group, with White men having the highest suicide rates and Black or African American women having the lowest suicide rates in the United States, as shown in the chart below. There are not much data currently available on ethnic group differences in suicidal thoughts and attempts among adults. This is worth noting because, as described above regarding men versus women, suicide attempts and suicidal thoughts can occur in patterns that look quite different from suicide deaths. In recent years, there has been a reported increase in suicide attempts among Black or African American adolescents (Lindsey et al., 2019), and Black or African American children were more likely to die by suicide than White children (Bridge et al., 2018). These findings highlight the importance of considering age and other factors for a fuller picture of the people most afflicted by suicidal thoughts and behaviors (Opara et al., 2020).

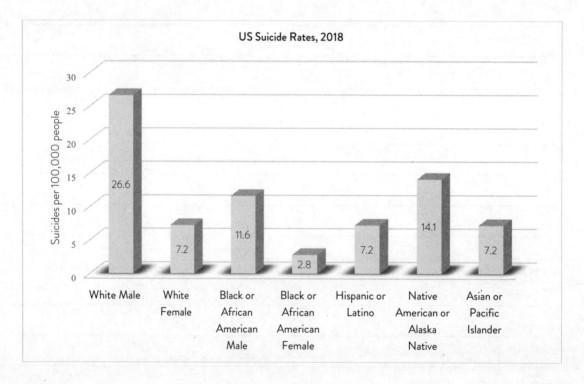

In 2018, the age groups most likely to die by suicide in the United States were middle-aged adults 45–64 years old (see chart on the next page; Drapeau and McIntosh, 2020). There are also surveys that gather information about differences in suicidal thoughts and behaviors across age groups. A 2016 national survey of US adults estimated that 4 percent (9.8 million) had seriously considered suicide in the past year. Of those who considered suicide, approximately 13 percent (1.3 million) went on to attempt it (Substance Abuse and Mental Health Services Administration, 2017). Suicidal thoughts and attempts in the previous year were more common among younger adults (ages 18–25) than any other age group (8.8 percent seriously considered suicide and 1.8 percent attempted suicide), but older adults were much more likely to die by suicide than younger people when they attempted it (Drapeau and McIntosh, 2020).

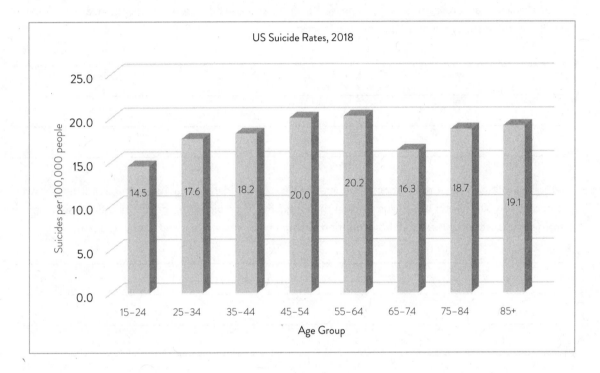

Research also suggests that lesbian, gay, bisexual, and transgender (LGBT) people report higher rates of suicidal thoughts and attempts as compared to cisgender, heterosexual people (e.g., Hottes et al., 2016; Marshall et al., 2015). More research is needed on the nature of these disparities, but the existing literature points to LGBT people facing greater discrimination both at systemic (e.g., difficulty accessing affirming medical care) and individual (e.g., higher rates of bullying) levels as a cause of the disparity (e.g., Salway et al., 2019; Testa et al., 2017). It's important to note that, despite the higher rates, many LGBT people do not have suicidal thoughts and that equal rights are linked to lower risk. For example, Raifman and colleagues (2017) found that state implementation of same-sex marriage policies was linked to a decrease in suicide attempts among LGBT adolescents. If you are interested in additional mental health resources specifically designed for LGBT people, please see appendix B.

Now, let's explore how your cultural experiences have impacted your own suicidal thoughts. I want to create a clearer context for you to place your experiences in, because that will help point you to effective coping strategies that best fit your life.

Experiences of Discrimination and Sources of Strength Connected to My Identity

Have you experienced discrimination, prejudice, or mistreatment that is linked to your suicidal thoughts? For example, have you been bullied, teased, or excluded from a job, housing, or medical care because of your ethnicity, race, religion, disability, age, sexual orientation, gender identity, weight, income, education level, veteran status, or another part of your identity?

_____

_____

_____

_____

Are there cultural values, rituals, or communities related to your identity that have served as strengths when it comes to your mental health and suicidal thoughts? For example, some people find pride and support from spiritual communities, LGBT organizations, refugee cultural centers, and family traditions.

_____

_____

_____

_____

You did outstanding work exploring those influences on your mental health! With each step, you are getting closer to understanding yourself and your mental health needs.

What Is Nonsuicidal Self-Injury?

If you have not engaged in NSSI, you can skip this section and go right to the next: "Encouraging Self-Statements." This workbook will not go into depth about NSSI, since its focus is on suicidal thoughts and behaviors. I'm including basic NSSI information here because suicidal thoughts and NSSI behaviors are related and because people who harm themselves are at higher risk for suicide attempts (Klonsky et al., 2013).

Burning, cutting, and scratching yourself are the most common types of NSSI, but there are other methods people use too. Anyone can be affected by NSSI, but adolescents and young adults seem at highest risk for it (International Society for the Study of Self-Injury, 2019). An estimated 17.2 percent of teenagers, 13.4 percent of young adults, and 5.5 percent of adults report that they have intentionally hurt themselves at least once in their lives (Swannell et al., 2014). If you ever intentionally hurt yourself, what was the reason? If it was to lessen painful emotions, then you are in the same boat as most people who hurt themselves. Other reasons people hurt themselves include punishing themselves, trying to communicate something to others, or trying to feel something other than numbness (Bentley et al., 2014; Klonsky, 2007).

There are probably different reasons that NSSI and suicide risk are linked, but the most important ones to understand are the ones that are relevant to you. Let's take some time to explore this in the next section, but first let's check in. Are you hanging in there with the different topics I'm asking you to think about? Remember that it's okay to take a break when you need one. It might be a good time to process how you're feeling in your journal or to do a calming activity. Make sure to remind yourself that this process is work and that every step you take is a reason to feel proud.

The Role of Nonsuicidal Self-Injury

At what age did you first engage in NSSI? _____

How old were you the most recent time you engaged in NSSI? _____

How often do you have urges to engage in NSSI?

never	yearly or less	monthly	weekly	daily

What prompts your urges to engage in NSSI?

Emotions (e.g., sadness, anger, loneliness, shame, boredom, numbness, fear, jealousy):

_____

_____

Interpersonal situations (e.g., fighting with people, feeling excluded or rejected, being asked to do something you don't want to do):

_____

_____

Stressors (e.g., painful memories, trauma flashbacks, hard day at work or school, worry):

_____

_____

How do you cope with those urges (e.g., distraction, exercise, take a shower, call a friend, journal)?

_____

_____

Do you already understand how NSSI is related to your suicidal thoughts and behavior? If not, you can use this list as a way to start figuring it out.

☐ It's a sign that my suicide risk is high.

☐ It gives me some escape from emotional pain without ending my life.

☐ It shows others that I need their help.

☐ It shows others that I'm in pain.

☐ It means that my mental health is getting worse.

☐ It's unrelated to my suicide risk.

☐ It means that my stress levels are high.

☐ It means that I'm less in control of my behaviors than usual.

☐ Other: _____

Sometimes exploring these feelings can bring up shame, guilt, or blame. I hope that this doesn't happen for you, but in our darkest moments, self-compassion and acceptance can be especially hard to come by. In the exercise below, I have listed some self-statements to counter any self-judgment you might feel. In addition to reading these statements, you can also try imagining someone who loves you embracing you with warmth and empathy. I encourage you to seek support from people who remind you of your worth as you process painful emotions. In chapter 6, we'll spend more time on strategies for increasing self-compassion.

Encouraging Self-Statements

☐ It's understandable that I would feel this way after what I've been through.

☐ It's unfair to be discriminated against because of who I am, which is why I should be extra kind to myself in the face of it.

☐ Other people might question the validity of my experiences. That doesn't mean that they're right or that there is something wrong with me.

☐ When I'm in pain, it makes sense that I think about ways to find relief.

☐ I'm not alone in feeling suicidal. There are other people out there struggling.

☐ My struggle with emotional pain is not a sign that I am weak, have a character flaw, or am a bad person.

☐ In the past, I did the best I could with the information I had at the time.

☐ I can work on change while treating myself in a kind, loving manner.

☐ I am worthy of kindness and wellness.

☐ Even if others suggest that I'm to blame for my suicidal thoughts, that does not mean that they're right.

☐ People have a hard time understanding suicidal thoughts, but that doesn't mean that their opinions about me and my life are true.

☐ I can dislike my feelings and parts of my life without disliking myself.

☐ I am capable of learning new ways to cope with my pain.

☐ Other: _____

☐ Other: _____

☐ Other: _____

I hope that this chapter helped you identify some of the specific types of stressors leading to your suicidal thoughts and behaviors and the environments that they exist in. I want to thank you for taking the time and effort to work through these issues with me. You are worth the investment you're putting into this workbook! In the next chapter, we'll go into more depth about the causes of suicidal desire before focusing on tools to address them.

Summary of Key Points

- Sometimes people respond to suicidal thoughts in ways that feel bad. That doesn't mean that you're wrong for seeking support.

- Certain people are at higher risk for suicide than others, in part due to societal factors. Understanding yourself and the impact of your environment are steps toward creating an effective mental health plan that is tailored to your personal needs.

- You are not alone in your struggles. There are reasons to be hopeful. If shame comes up as you work through this book, try approaching yourself with self-compassion instead of self-criticism.

Reflection

What thoughts, ideas, and feelings did you have while reading and working through this chapter? Were there certain parts you didn't relate to? What parts did you relate to most? What did you learn?

CHAPTER 3

Uncover Causes

Now that you have a deeper understanding of your suicidal thoughts, let's uncover the causes. Through research, scientists have identified factors that are linked to higher risk for suicide (Franklin et al., 2017; O'Conner and Nock, 2014; Van Orden et al., 2010). The chapter will begin by exploring how ten of these risk factors affect you. After that, we'll take a closer look at the 3ST mentioned in chapter 1 and see how the theory applies to your life (Klonsky and May, 2015). The purpose of this chapter is to increase awareness about the causes of your suicidal thoughts, which will help you make the most out of the other chapters in this workbook.

Risk Factors That Affect Me

This worksheet lists ten risk factors from Van Orden et al. (2010): mental illness(es), previous suicide attempt(s), social isolation, physical illness, unemployment, family conflict, impulsivity, childhood abuse, combat exposure, and family history of suicide. For each one that applies to you, write how it affects your suicidal thoughts right now. If it does not affect you currently but did in the past, please note that as well. If the risk factor doesn't apply to you, skip that section. To guide you through this, I provided examples.

Mental Illness

Mental illnesses or health problems that I currently struggle with: posttraumatic stress disorder after being sexually assaulted, panic attacks, drink too much sometimes

How they affect me now: I have trouble sleeping. I didn't trust people for a long time after the sexual assault. Sometimes I have flashbacks when my partner touches me, and that sets me off for a whole day. The panic attacks scare me and make it harder to try going out to new places. When I use alcohol, it goes one of two ways: creates an escape from my problems or makes them bigger. I can't tell which one it's going to be ahead of time. Sometimes I feel broken because I have to deal with all of this, and that feeling prompts suicidal thoughts.

Mental Illness(es)

Mental illnesses or health problems that I currently struggle with: _____

_____

How they affect me now: _____

_____

_____

Previous Suicide Attempt(s)

How it affects me now: I attempted suicide when I was a teenager and was being bullied at school. It doesn't affect me much now except that it's a reminder to not let things get to that point. I don't want to go back to how I felt then.

Previous Suicide Attempt(s)

How it affects me now: _____

_____

_____

Social Isolation

How it affects me now: When I feel down, I push people away. I'm lucky to have a supportive family and a few close friends who check in on me though. I need to remember to reach out when I feel lonely instead of avoiding people. The suicidal thoughts definitely get worse when I spend a lot of time alone.

Social Isolation

How it affects me now: _____

_____

_____

Physical Illness

Physical illnesses or health problems I currently struggle with: I have diabetes, and when my blood sugar levels get too high or too low, it affects my mood.

How they affect me now: I get frustrated that I have to deal with something that most people don't have to deal with. It's an extra challenge in my life. Traveling is harder, and I feel anxious when my blood sugar goes too far up or too far down. This doesn't really affect my suicidal thoughts unless it happens at the same time as other stresses in my life.

Physical Illness

Physical illnesses or health problems I currently struggle with: _____

How they affect me now: _____

_____

_____

Unemployment

How it affects me now: I'm employed right now and like my job as a cook. If the restaurant's business is slow or the economy is bad, I sometimes worry I'll lose my job. That's happened to me before, and it gets me down. If I have a long period of unemployment, I start to feel like a burden, and that can lead to suicidal thoughts that people would be better off without me.

Unemployment

How it affects me now: _____

_____

_____

Family Conflict

How it affects me now: I get along well with my family except for my stepmom, but I don't talk to her or see her ever, so it doesn't affect me currently. I get upset if I think about the past, but for now, it doesn't bother me much. Sometimes when my twin babies are crying, and my husband and I are not getting along, I start to have thoughts about wishing I were dead, because I can't cope. It feels like too much to deal with at times. When things are good with my babies and husband, I feel happy and want to live for a long time.

Family Conflict

How it affects me now: _____

_____

_____

Impulsivity

How it affects me now: Sometimes when I'm upset, I spend too much money trying to make myself feel better. It works at first, but then I get more upset with myself and more worried about finances. This doesn't really lead to suicidal thoughts, but I do get really self-critical when it happens.

Impulsivity

How it affects me now: _____

_____

_____

Childhood Abuse

How it affects me now: Even though I have worked through it a lot, sometimes I feel like my feelings don't matter, because they didn't matter when I was a kid. Any time I was hurt, I was told that it was my fault for being a bad child. It makes me want to disappear until I can bring myself back to the present moment.

Childhood Abuse

How it affects me now: _____

_____

_____

Combat Exposure

How it affects me now: I did one tour of duty in Iraq and saw some horrible things. Sometimes, when I see people in military uniforms, it triggers flashbacks that make my mood feel off for a few days. I don't feel more suicidal, but I do feel more disconnected from life.

Combat Exposure

How it affects me now: _____

_____

_____

Family History of Suicide

How it affects me now: My brother died by suicide when I was a teenager. I still feel sad—like there's more I should have done to stop him. When I feel suicidal, I think about how I can't do that to my parents after they lost my brother. Their hearts were broken.

Family History of Suicide

How it affects me now: _____

_____

_____

The Three-Step Theory

Now that you have more insight into the specific factors that affect you, let's learn about how they can lead to suicidal thoughts and behaviors through the 3ST framework. As mentioned in chapter 2, many more people have thoughts about suicide than act on them. The 3ST framework will help you recognize if and when your thoughts are more likely to turn into suicidal action and require your crisis plan (detailed in chapter 4). Now let's explore each step of the 3ST.

Step 1: Pain and Hopelessness

If you are feeling pain and hopelessness, you might start considering suicide. That pain can be emotional, physical, or both. The 3ST says that the presence of pain alone does not cause suicidal desire unless you also feel hopeless about it changing in the future. The theory purposely doesn't specify the source of pain, because it all depends on your personal situation. With suicidal thoughts, some possible sources of pain include the end of an important relationship, the death of a loved one, illness, financial difficulties, job loss, feeling a lack of joy or purpose, or other stressors. Let's reflect on how step 1 applies to you.

What Causes My Pain?

Are you experiencing pain right now? Please use the space below to write about what your pain feels like and where it's coming from. Write freely about whatever comes to your mind—body sensations, thoughts, emotions—all of it belongs in the space below.

_____

_____

_____

_____

_____

_____

_____

_____

_____

_____

_____

_____

Thank you for writing about your pain. Some people find it helpful to write about their pain, while others find it difficult. Either way, I hope you feel proud of taking time to process it. Even if you're not exactly sure what it is, writing about what it feels like can shed light on useful ways to address it. Chapters 5 and 6 focus on reducing your emotional pain through problem solving, CBT, self-compassion, and acceptance.

Do I Feel Hopeless?

Do you feel hopeless? What does that feel like right now? Why do you feel that things won't get better? What would need to change for you to have more hope?

_____

_____

_____

_____

_____

_____

_____

_____

_____

_____

_____

Thank you for reflecting on hopelessness in your life. I am so sorry if you have been struggling with ways to find hope. Chapter 7 is all about increasing hope. Finding reasons for hope is not easy sometimes, but we will look for them together. When you feel hopeful, your suicidal thoughts don't feel as intense.

Step 2: Connections to Life

If your level of pain is so high that it overpowers the connections that make you want to live, your suicidal desire will become more intense. Connections to life can include people (e.g., friends, family, romantic partners) or other aspects of your life (e.g., jobs, projects, spirituality). If your connections make your life worth living, you will have more modest levels of suicidal desire.

My Connections to Life

When you have suicidal thoughts, what makes you decide to keep on living?

_____

Who are the people you feel most connected to?

_____

Are there others you're connected to that are not mentioned above (e.g., pets)?

_____

What parts of your life help you feel connected (e.g., a role, an activity, your spiritual beliefs)?

_____

_____

What do you find most meaningful in your life?

_____

_____

_____

_____

_____

_____

Thank you for exploring your feelings of connection and disconnection. It's tough to struggle with ways to find meaning and relationships that feel good to you. Chapter 8 helps with strengthening relationships and chapter 9 helps increase your sense of meaning and purpose. Fostering relationships and meaning can be challenging, but this workbook will walk you through it step by step.

Step 3: Capability for Suicide

Humans are born with strong survival instincts that draw us to life, push us away from pain, and urge us to protect ourselves in the face of harm. That means that most people who desire suicide will not attempt it, because of fears about pain and death. The third step of 3ST identifies three kinds of capability thought to be present in people who override this survival instinct and attempt suicide: (1) dispositional (e.g., genetics related to how sensitive you are to pain), (2) acquired (e.g., experiences you have that lower your fear of death and increase your pain tolerance, such as NSSI or other types of physically painful experiences), and (3) practical (e.g., having access to and knowledge of suicide methods).

My Capability for Suicide

Let's take some time to examine how these different parts of capability for suicide affect you. Are there certain things about your personality, your experiences, and your knowledge that influence your capability for suicide? Do you understand how to use certain methods for suicide? Do you have access to them currently? Are you the type of person who has a high pain tolerance and isn't afraid of death? Explore these questions in the space below.

_____

_____

_____

_____

_____

_____

Your responses to these questions deepen your understanding of your capability for suicide. The content in chapter 10 goes into more depth on ways to create emotional and physical safety. Chapter 10 also discusses ways to prevent increasing your capability for suicide.

I hope this chapter has helped you understand the causes of suicidal thoughts and behaviors in your life. Now that you are familiar with the 3ST framework and how it applies to your experiences, we'll move on to chapter 4 to learn about coping with crises.

Summary of Key Points

- People end up feeling suicidal through different, individual pathways in their lives.

- People tend to share certain types of common experiences when they are feeling suicidal. Science has helped to identify them.

- The 3ST proposes that:
  - Pain and hopelessness lead to suicidal desire.

  - When your connections to life are stronger than your pain, modest suicidal desire develops. If your pain exceeds your connections to life, strong suicidal desire develops.

  - If someone has strong suicidal desire and the capability for suicide, they are at risk for attempting suicide.

Reflection

What thoughts, ideas, and feelings did you have while reading and working through this chapter? Were there certain parts you didn't relate to? What parts did you relate to most? What did you learn?

CHAPTER 4

Cope with Crises

As a therapist, I know that long-term suffering takes a toll on people. I wrote this workbook because I want to teach you strategies that alleviate the pain in your life. Even though you're suffering, the fact that you're reading this workbook tells me that some part of you wants to be alive. I'm grateful for that, because your life is important. No one else has the unique qualities and gifts that you bring to the world. Before we dive deeper into causes and ways to address your pain, let's make a plan for keeping you safe through suicidal crises. First we'll talk about how to know whether you are in a crisis, meaning that you are in a dangerous state and are likely to hurt yourself. Next we'll work together to develop a plan for safe and healthy coping, including seeking support from others and identifying ways to lessen your pain. Even if your suicidal thoughts tend to be mostly passive, it is useful to develop a crisis plan so that you're prepared if that changes.

Am I in Crisis?

When you're in intense pain, it can turn into a crisis. Each person has their own signs that their suicide risk is getting to a dangerous spot. Research has identified some of the most common ones (insomnia, nightmares, sudden unintentional weight loss, agitation, social withdrawal; Chu et al., 2015), but it's important that we figure out the ones that tend to be specifically true for you. Let's start with an example and then work together to identify signs that a crisis is developing.

Diana has dealt with depression on and off since she was fifteen. She's now thirty-six and has learned new coping skills in therapy and developed close friendships. Most days, she feels good and does not have thoughts about killing herself. However, she finds that the thoughts return when she's experiencing something highly stressful (e.g., a fight with her partner, a conflict at work) or has had many stressors in a row (e.g., sickness, unexpected bills to pay).

Recently, she received feedback about her job performance. Overall, the review was positive, but she couldn't stop focusing on the criticism that she needed to improve the timeliness for completing projects. Diana found that she was ruminating about her evaluation throughout the day and that made it hard to focus on her work. She went home and talked to her partner about it, seeking reassurance. At first, the reassurance helped, but then it started to wear off by bedtime. In the days that followed, she repeatedly sought reassurance from him, and it helped less and less. She struggled to fall asleep, as her mind was filled with thoughts about how she was not a worthy person and fears that she would lose her job because of it.

Diana became convinced that she messed up her chances to succeed in her career. Her partner started expressing frustration that this was going on for weeks, and she worried that he would leave her. She began distancing herself from him and her coworkers. She was on edge, filled with shame, and started thinking about killing herself to escape the constant worry and guilt. Diana began thinking about overdosing on her prescribed medications after her partner went to work the following day.

There are several signs that a crisis is developing for Diana. The sad and shameful mood that is persisting for days has disrupted her sleep, her work, and her relationship. She is starting to spiral into a dangerous pattern, one that she has experienced before and that once led to a suicide attempt. Her mind is jumping around to different ways to make the pain stop. This is especially risky, because she's considering specific plans for how she will hurt herself.

What are the signs that you're in a crisis? The worksheet below will guide you through the process of identifying them, with Diana's experiences used as examples.

Signs That I'm in Crisis (Diana's Example)

- ☐ nightmares

- ☑ insomnia (can't fall asleep or can't stay asleep)

- ☑ social withdrawal (e.g., not answering texts, canceling plans)

- ☑ self-hatred, shame

- ☐ feeling hopeless

- ☑ feeling agitated, restless

- ☑ thinking about killing myself a lot more than usual

- ☑ planning for suicide (e.g., getting a gun, thinking about when I might do it)

- ☐ not taking care of myself (e.g., stop showering, not eating enough food)

- ☑ I feel like I hate myself and it lasts more than a day.

- ☑ I overthink—especially at bedtime.

- ☑ I avoid people.

- ☑ I imagine ending my life.

- ☑ I start thinking that other people would be better off without me.

- ☑ I don't think things will ever get better.

Signs That I'm in Crisis

Check off the warning signs that apply to you, and then please add your own, if you think of others.

- ☐ nightmares

- ☐ insomnia (can't fall asleep or can't stay asleep)

- ☐ social withdrawal (e.g., not answering texts, canceling plans)

- ☐ self-hatred, shame

- ☐ feeling hopeless

- ☐ feeling agitated, restless

- ☐ thinking about killing myself a lot more than usual

- ☐ planning for suicide (e.g., getting a gun, thinking about when I might do it)

- ☐ not taking care of myself (e.g., stop showering, not eating enough food)

- ☐ _____

- ☐ _____

- ☐ _____

- ☐ _____

- ☐ _____

- ☐ _____

Great job taking the time to fill that out! It can be so painful to remember times when you were in crisis. I appreciate you thinking about your warning signs even though it may hurt to think back on those times. This kind of reflection will help keep you safe in the future.

How Can I Quickly Reduce the Intensity of My Emotional Pain?

When you're in a crisis, you might feel agitated, sad, or a mix of different uncomfortable emotions. If you want to kill yourself, it's probably because your pain is so intense that death feels like the only way to find relief. That is why it's important to find other ways to relieve the pain. This workbook will go into greater depth about reducing your longer-term emotional pain in the next two chapters. For now, let's come up with a list of go-to strategies that quickly reduce the sense of urgency to hurt yourself that arises during a crisis.

Every person has certain activities that work best for them, but generally, the following activities have the most impact:

- **things that absorb a lot of your attention**
  - an engrossing movie, book, or show
  - video games
  - building something
  - creating art or coloring
  - working on a house project
  - cooking or baking
  - working on puzzles
  - talking with a friend
  - a change of scenery
  - cleaning or organizing

- **things that influence you physically in a positive way**
  - exercise
  - a hot bath or shower
  - splashing cold water on your face
  - taking deep breaths
  - playing a sport
  - drinking hot tea
  - getting a massage
  - stretching
  - tensing and relaxing your muscles
  - changing into comfortable clothes

- **things that evoke positive feelings**
  - looking at space, nature, or animal pictures
  - singing or dancing to a song you love
  - listening to live music

- hugging a loved one
- spending time with a pet
- looking through pictures of family or friends
- lighting a scented candle
- going to sit somewhere with beautiful scenery
- eating a favorite food
- watching stand-up comedy

We'll start with Diana's activities as an example before we get to your list. The goal of this exercise is to come up with a variety of activities, so that there will always be some that you can do at any time and any place. For example, if you like to go on long walks, you might not be able to when it's raining or dark outside, and taking a long bath might be comforting, but you typically can't do that at work or while driving. Having a range of options will prevent you from feeling stuck.

Ten Ways to Reduce Emotional Pain (Diana's Example)

1. go for a walk

2. take a hot shower

3. play a game on my phone

4. take a bubble bath

5. splash cold water on my face

6. do a deep-breathing exercise

7. play loud, soothing music

8. drink herbal tea

9. sit outside in the sun

10. watch a funny movie

Now that you have read Diana's example, try to think of ten ways that you can decrease intense emotional pain during a crisis.

Ten Ways to Reduce Emotional Pain

1. _____

2. _____

3. _____

4. _____

5. _____

6. _____

7. _____

8. _____

9. _____

10. _____

A Note on Insomnia and Nightmares

I mentioned above that insomnia and nightmares can both be warning signs for suicide (Liu et al., 2020). In appendix B, I suggest some in-depth workbooks that specifically help with sleep troubles (Silberman, 2008). In this section, I'll share some basic tips:

- One of the most common and unhelpful reactions to sleep difficulty is to "castastrophize," or start thinking about the worst-case scenario of any situation—in this case, thinking that you'll never fall asleep and how bad tomorrow will be for you. This raises your anxiety and can even cause panic, which makes it harder to sleep. I know it's difficult, but try to remind yourself that while it would be nice to sleep, it's not a disaster if you can't fall asleep. Aim for rest and relaxation, which are also restorative.

- If you don't fall asleep after a while, try getting up to read or listen to a somewhat boring book or to do an activity that is not physically strenuous (e.g., fold laundry or reorganize a small area of your home, like a desktop or shelf). Getting out of your bed when you can't fall asleep helps prevent an association between your bed and frustration.

- Regularize your sleep pattern: get up at the same time every morning—even if you had trouble sleeping the night before—and eliminate afternoon naps. This can make it easier to fall asleep at night.

- Try relaxing routines to wind down before bed (e.g., a bubble bath, shower, prayer, reading a book, talking with someone about your day, doing a relaxation exercise) and avoid stimulating activities (e.g., social media feeds, news stories, intense exercise).

- Limit your caffeine intake, especially in the evening.

- Try adding some exercise into your day, but make sure it's not too close to bedtime.

- Consider reaching out to a mental health professional for CBT for insomnia, which is effective (Boness et al., 2020).

For nightmares, you can also seek help from a mental health professional. You may want to ask about a science-informed treatment called image rehearsal therapy, which reduces nightmares (Krakow and Zadra, 2010). Briefly, image rehearsal therapy works by writing out your nightmares, changing the endings to happy ones, and imagining the new endings.

Who Can I Ask for Help?

Let's think about who can support you, so that you don't have go through this alone. Finding help is important, because it reduces the pressure to figure everything out on your own. When at least one other person is helping you out, the crisis feels more manageable. Connecting with others in your time of need can also prevent the extra pain of loneliness on top of your suffering.

People Who Can Help When I'm in Crisis (Diana's Example)

Who lifts my spirits?

friends:	how they can help me:
Steven	tell me a funny story or joke
Marigold	remind me that I've made it through tough times before
Inez	share encouraging words

family members:

Dad	tell me that he believes in me and loves me
David	talk about funny memories we have together
Mamie	hang out and play video games

others (e.g., partner, coworker, neighbor):

André	cook a meal or go for a walk together, give me a hug
Sumie	gossip about silly stuff at work
Arun	drink coffee or tea together

Who is there when I want to share my feelings?

name:	how they can help me:
Elizabeth	listen to me without giving advice
André	listen and show confidence in me
Pastor Leta	share advice and religious wisdom, point me to prayers that will help

Who can help me with coping skills and safety (e.g., therapists and other professional help, family members and friends)?

name:	how they can help me:
Dr. Bernal	guide me through coping skills
Crisis Text Line	text with me until my feelings are less intense and I have a safety plan in place
Mom	come over until the intense feelings pass, hold on to my medications until I'm not in crisis anymore, keep me company until I feel better

Now fill out your own worksheet. Please list people who can support you during a crisis. The goal is to name at least one person for each category. If you get stuck on one of the categories, move to the next one. You can always come back to it. For each person or resource, please make sure their phone number is programmed into your phone and that you specifically list how they can help you. When you're in a crisis, it can be hard to think about what you need. If you plan now, you can reference this worksheet during those hard times. It can be helpful to contact the people on your list and ask them if they can be part of your safety plan. If you let them know how they can help ahead of time, it might make things easier in your moment of need. You may not feel comfortable discussing all of the details with some of the people you have listed, and that is okay too. (A downloadable copy of this worksheet is available on the New Harbinger website, so you can also print it out and have it ready in a convenient place: http://www.newharbinger.com/47025.)

People Who Can Help When I'm in Crisis

Who lifts my spirits?

friends: how they can help me:

_____   _____

_____   _____

_____   _____

family members:

_____   _____

_____   _____

_____   _____

others (e.g., partner, coworker, neighbor):

_____   _____

_____   _____

_____   _____

Who is there when I want to share my feelings?

name: how they can help me:

_____   _____

_____   _____

_____   _____

Who can help me with coping skills and safety (e.g., therapists and other professional help, family members and friends)?

name: how they can help me:

_____   _____

_____   _____

_____   _____

Do you feel comfortable asking people for help when you're struggling? If not, take a moment to think about what gets in the way of seeking support when you're in crisis. Maybe you have had bad experiences before or you're not sure that you're worthy of help. As a reminder, your life is valuable, and you are worthy of support, even if you don't feel that way right now. If you're not sure how to start a conversation about needing support, read through the suggestions in the exercise below.

How to Ask for Help

Circle the statements that you would feel comfortable using and add any other phrasing or sentences that you think of on your own.

- I'm feeling pretty down right now. Would it be okay for me to talk to you about it?

- I'm struggling right now. Can you help me come up with ways to get help?

- I'm thinking about hurting myself, and it worries me. I think I'll feel better if someone listens to me or spends some time with me. Can we meet for lunch or go for a walk?

- I'm worried I might hurt myself. Would you hold on to my prescription pills until I'm feeling better?

- It's hard for me to ask for help, but I think I'm in crisis right now. Will you keep me company while I figure out how to handle this?

- _____

- _____

- _____

- _____

- _____

How Can I Keep Myself Safe?

If you're in a suicidal crisis, you are more likely to attempt suicide if you have access to suicide methods (e.g., a gun, pills to overdose on). That means that you can increase your safety during a crisis by putting distance between you and methods for hurting yourself. For example, research shows that owning a gun increases suicide risk, and that it's probably due to access to a dangerous method during points of intense suicidal desire (Anestis and Houtsma, 2017). Reducing your access to these methods during crises can be lifesaving (e.g., storing your ammunition separately from your gun, locking your gun in a safe), because the most intense suicidal desire tends to decrease over the period of time that it would take to access that method (Anestis, 2018).

With Diana's example, she is thinking about overdosing on her prescribed medications. Part of Diana's crisis plan could involve asking a relative or friend to store the medication at their home so that she doesn't have it in her own home. She can stop by when she needs it, and they can give her only the prescribed amount. Or she could keep it in a lockbox that only her partner has the combination to, or she could ask the prescriber to reduce the number of pills she gets each time. You might be thinking, _If you take away that method, I'll just use another one._ I have heard many people bring up this understandable concern. However, research shows that it's often not the case that people seek out another method if they don't have access to their preferred one (Zalsman et al., 2016). In addition, sometimes the other method is a less dangerous method than the first, and thus lives can be saved that way as well. That is hopeful news, because it means that there are clear ways to keep yourself safe. Let's explore the specifics of your safety plan with the worksheet below.

Staying Safe

Do you have any guns in your home?

yes   no

How can you create safety when you are in crisis?

☐ store guns outside of my home (e.g., someone else's house)

☐ keep bullets separate from my gun

☐ store gun safely (e.g., in a locked safe)

Are there other methods you have been thinking of using to hurt yourself? List each one below.

_____

_____

How can you make yourself safer by reducing access to these methods? Ask someone for help (e.g., a therapist, a friend, call a crisis hotline) if you are unsure how to fill this out.

_____

_____

Who Can I Contact in an Emergency?

Your life is so important, and I want you to stay with us. If you're experiencing one or more of these signs of high suicide risk, please consider contacting one of the emergency services listed in the next section (Stanley et al., 2016):

- You feel like you can't stop yourself from suicide.

- Your mind is not clear enough to think through alternatives to suicide.

- Your suicidal desire is building with intensity over time.

- You have a specific plan and intend to act on it.

- You feel agitated, like you're going to "crawl out of your skin."

- You feel intense disgust with others or yourself (e.g., that others would be better off without you, that you should withdraw from everyone).

- You have lost hope that your life will get better.

- You can't think of anyone who can stay with you while you are in crisis.

Below I have listed organizations as suggestions for you, but please look up the current phone numbers for them (most should be easily available through an internet search or by asking a medical or mental health professional) and fill in the blanks. Please add any additional emergency numbers that you can contact and then program them all into your phone so that they are there whenever you need them. (A copy of this list is available on the New Harbinger website, so you can also print it out and have it ready in a convenient place: http://www.newharbinger.com/47025.)

Emergency Services I Can Contact to Stay Safe

1. National Suicide Prevention Lifeline   phone #: _____

2. Crisis Text Line   phone #: _____

3. Walk-In Clinic   phone #: _____

    address: _____

    _____

4. Other Emergency Lines (e.g., hotlines, warmlines)   phone #: _____

    phone #: _____

5. Mobile Mental Health Crisis Unit(s)   phone #: _____

    phone #: _____

6. Local Emergency Room   phone #: _____

    address: _____

    _____

7. Others:

_____

_____

_____

Make Your Crisis Plan Easy to Access

If you have made it this far into the chapter, that means you're doing a wonderful job planning for coping during suicidal crises. Now that we have gone through each step in depth, let's tie them together into a single page summary. This one-page crisis plan is designed so that you can access it at all times. You can tear out the page and keep it in your wallet, place it somewhere prominent in your house like your refrigerator, or take a picture of it with your phone. The key is to make it so you can easily look at it whenever you need it. In addition to keeping at least one copy of the plan with you at all times, I recommend sharing it with others you trust (e.g., your therapist, a close friend, a partner) so that they can support you in a crisis situation. If they have a copy, they will be able to follow the instructions to provide you with the support that you need.

The summary of your crisis plan also asks you to list your top reasons for living. When you're feeling suicidal, it can be hard to remember why you want to stay alive. The list will make it easier to think about when the suicidal thoughts come into your mind. I hope you find this chapter helpful for staying safe during a crisis. The world is a better place with you in it.

My Crisis Plan Summary (Diana's Example)

Signs that I am in crisis: insomnia, planning how I will kill myself, withdrawing from my partner and friends, losing hope, feeling "on edge"

Reasons why I want to live: I want to go on that trip I have planned. I don't want my parents to be heartbroken. I want to celebrate my fortieth birthday.

People I can contact (make sure you program their numbers into your phone)

Lift my spirits: Steven, Marigold, Inez, Dad, David, Mamie, Sumie, Arun, André

Share my feelings: Elizabeth, André, Pastor Leta

Get advice for coping and safety: Dr. Bernal, Crisis Text Line, Mom

Ways to keep myself safe: ask my partner to hold on to my medications

Ways to rapidly reduce intense emotional pain: go for a long walk, take a hot shower, play a game on my phone, take a bubble bath, splash cold water on my face, do a breathing exercise, drink herbal tea, sit outside in the sun, watch a funny movie

Emergency numbers and locations:

National Suicide Prevention Lifeline   Emergency Room Closest to Me

Mobile Mental Health Crisis Unit

After reading through Diana's example, fill out your crisis plan in the worksheet below.

My Crisis Plan Summary

Signs that I am in crisis: _____

_____

Reasons why I want to live: _____

_____

People I can contact (make sure you program their numbers into your phone)

    Lift my spirits: _____

    Share my feelings: _____

    Get advice for coping and safety: _____

Ways to keep myself safe: _____

Ways to rapidly reduce intense emotional pain: _____

_____

_____

Emergency numbers and locations:

_____

_____

_____

Summary of Key Points

- Each person has their own signs that they are entering into a crisis. It's important to identify what yours tend to be so that you know when to use your crisis plan.

- Powerful strategies for reducing the intensity of suicidal crises include getting support from others, reducing access to suicide methods, safe options for reducing emotional pain, and having access to emergency numbers.

- It's hard to address problems when you're in the middle of a crisis. Having your plan available will make it easier to stay safe.

Reflection

What thoughts, ideas, and feelings did you have while reading and working through this chapter? Were there certain parts you didn't relate to? What parts did you relate to most? What did you learn?

CHAPTER 5

Reduce Emotional Pain

Most people think about suicide when they're in so much emotional pain that life feels excruciating. Because you're reading this book, I imagine that you have felt that kind of pain. I'm sorry that you have been in such a dark place, and I'm grateful that you're still here. Your life matters, and so does your well-being. Suicide prevention isn't just about keeping you from killing yourself; it's also about creating a life that feels good and meaningful so that you want to stay alive. In this chapter, you'll learn how to identify the sources of your pain and decrease it through problem solving and CBT strategies.

What Are the Causes of My Pain?

Many different types of situations can lead to emotional pain. Sometimes the sources of pain start to blur together and lead to an overall feeling of dread. When there is a general sense that life hurts, it can be particularly hard to pinpoint what you can do to feel better. It's helpful to start by getting specific about what's hurting you. Naming where your pain comes from will lead to the next step, which is finding effective ways to reduce it.

Different Parts of My Pain

In the space below, list sources of your emotional pain—no matter how big or small. Don't hold back or dismiss your feelings because you think they're not valid or important enough. This is a space for you to reflect on what's hurting without any judgment. Let's start with an example to guide you through the exercise.

> *After ten years of marriage, Javier found out that his husband, Dan, had cheated on him. Javier was hurt but still loved Dan. They entered couples therapy in an effort to resolve their problems. After six months, Dan decided that he wanted a divorce, because he was no longer in love with Javier. Javier's heart was broken. He became depressed and started thinking about ending his life.*

If Javier were completing this exercise, he might identify the following sources of emotional pain:

- I miss Dan.

- My dream of growing old with Dan is shattered.

- I blame myself for Dan cheating on me. I should have been a better husband.

- I'll be alone for the rest of my life. That was my one shot at happiness.

- All my friends think I'm a loser.

- I'm not going to be able to afford my apartment on my own.

Now, create your own list in the space below. It can be tough to name the things that cause us pain, but I know you can do it. You're stronger than you think.

- _____

- _____

- _____

- _____

- _____

- _____

- _____

- _____

- _____

Be Kind to Yourself as You Explore Emotional Pain

You took the first step toward decreasing your emotional pain by identifying the sources of it. I hope you feel proud of that. Now let's focus on responding to pain and explore those sources in more depth.

Normally, when we start thinking about hurtful parts of our lives, we may try to distract ourselves or otherwise avoid thinking about them. This is completely understandable. We don't want to turn our attention toward things that hurt. However, our brains are built to pay attention to pain, so it's difficult to take our minds off of it completely. This drives some people to use short-term behaviors such as drugs, alcohol, or avoidance to take their mind off the pain. Still, it lingers beneath the surface and has an impact once those distractions wear off.

A more effective and long-term strategy for reducing pain is to identify it, face it, and work through it. That means accepting the existence of pain rather than trying to talk yourself out of it or ignore it. At first, it can feel overwhelming to sit with your emotions. That is why it's important to validate your emotions and approach yourself like you would a friend, with kindness and patience.

First, try to find a quiet space where you can be without interruption. Then allow yourself to explore the painful sources you listed above. As each thought comes into your mind, you might have the urge to push it away. That is okay and makes sense, but what I'd like you to do is welcome those thoughts as opportunities to learn more about yourself instead of acting on that urge. Let go of judging yourself for the feelings you're having. Allow yourself to experience them without shame. If you start to judge yourself or think things like, *That's silly,* or *I should just get over it,* try these responses instead: *My pain is valid,* or *It's sad that I'm suffering.* Try talking to yourself like you would to a loved one expressing their troubles to you. Try to extend that loving manner to yourself. It might seem hard at first, but it gets easier with repeated, intentional practice.

Now imagine each source of pain in your mind and let yourself dig deep into the hurt, with the goal of gaining more understanding of yourself. If you need to take breaks, that's okay. There is no need to rush this process. No matter how you feel (numb, sad, angry) or how you react (tears, laughter, surprise), your feelings are okay to have. After you have spent time reflecting on the emotional pain you're feeling, set some time aside to write about what you learned. If you struggled with the self-compassion and acceptance suggestions, don't worry about that right now. Chapter 6 explores self-compassion and acceptance in more depth. For now, as you write about your pain, don't hold back at all. Write whatever comes to your mind. Don't worry about spelling or grammar or any technicalities. The purpose is just to express your feelings.

If you feel too overwhelmed after reading through the instructions above, try these other approaches:

- Set a time limit. Plan to only spend ten minutes thinking about emotional pain before taking a break to do something else. You can break up the task over a few days if that feels better.

- Plan to do something relaxing after completing the exercise (e.g., call a friend, go for a walk, listen to your favorite song).

- Encourage yourself by acknowledging that it's difficult but that you can do it. It is an important step toward feeling better.

How Can I Change My Situation Through Problem Solving?

Once you have labeled the sources of your emotional pain, there are different approaches to decrease it. Major options include: (1) changing the situation, (2) changing your view of the situation, or (3) a combination of options one and two (this applies to most situations). Let's begin by looking at ways to change the situation through the three steps of the problem-solving process:

1. Define the problem.

2. Brainstorm all possible solutions to the problem.

3. Select the best solution(s) and take action.

Define the Problem

Let's go through each step, using Javier's situation as an example. In order to define the problem, look at your list of sources of emotional pain and start with one that you have some influence over. From Javier's list, a good choice would be: *I'm not going to be able to afford my apartment on my own.* Now let's define the problem by adding details and clarifying what is most painful. Javier might define the problem more clearly as: *Dan and I used to share expenses. Now that he's moved out, I will have a hard time paying the rent and utility bills for the apartment on my income. I'm scared that I'll get evicted.*

Step 1: Define Your Problem

Define your problem below and be as specific as possible. Start with one of the items on your list of sources of emotional pain. After you work through the first problem, you can select the next one and try problem solving for that one. Get specific about the sources of your distress and remember to be gentle with yourself throughout the exercise.

_____

_____

_____

_____

_____

Excellent job being precise about the problem you are facing! Let's move on to the second step.

Brainstorm Possible Solutions

Creating a clearer picture of the problem is useful for finding possible solutions, which is the second step of the problem-solving process. When you're hurting, it's hard to see solutions. Try not to get frustrated with yourself if you feel stuck. Just do the best that you can and list any ideas that come to your mind—no matter how unrealistic they might seem at first. Also consider asking a friend, therapist, or some other trusted person to help you come up with solutions so you don't have to do it on your own. Here is what Javier came up with for the second step:

- Move into another, less expensive apartment.
  - I doubt I can break my lease early.
  - If it looks like I won't be able to cover my rent, I could ask for extra time and explain my circumstances.

★ - Get a better-paying job.
  - I can start looking, but it will probably take a while for this to happen. This doesn't solve my problem in the short term.

★ - Ask for a raise.
  - I will work up the nerve to try this. The worst that can happen is that they say no.

- Get a second job.
  - Pro: Could meet new people and stay busy (maybe think about Dan less).
  - Con: Could add extra stress, and I'm already struggling.

★ - Try to find a roommate.
  - Tiana mentioned that she had a friend who was looking for a new place to live.

- Ask Mom for a loan.
  - Sometimes, Mom holds favors like this over my head. Probably best to leave this as a last resort.

- Ask the bank for a loan.
  - I can try this if the other things don't work. I'd rather not take on more debt right now.

★ - Cut back on other expenses by being more careful with budgeting.
  - I could cut back on how much I go out to eat or order takeout. That would save some money. I could be more frugal when I'm buying clothes and other things.

★ - See a financial advisor through the Employee Assistance Program at work.
  - This is a good idea. It's free, and I might get some useful tips.

- Sell my guitar for extra cash.
  - I hope it doesn't come to this. My guitar helps me cope with my feelings. Playing music feels good and lifts my spirits.

After making the list, you can go through it and make notes about the pros, cons, obstacles, or other practical points of each proposed solution. For example, Javier noted that a downside of getting a second job could be adding stress at a time when he is struggling with his mental health. He also stated that selling his guitar is a bad idea right now because it helps him cope with his feelings in a positive way. On the other hand, Javier noted that there is no harm in asking for a raise, trying to find a roommate, and seeking help from a financial advisor. In addition, Javier thinks that he could cut some of his expenses. He put a star by each solution that seemed like one he could act on.

Javier came up with ten possible solutions, but there's no reason to feel bad if you come up with less. The number of solutions depends on your specific circumstances. The goal is to see whether there is something within your power that you can do to change the situation. Coming up with two or three possible solutions may be all that you need. I know this can be difficult, but you're doing a great job so far!

Step 2: Brainstorm Possible Solutions

In this step, write any possible solutions that come to mind. During the brainstorming period, I encourage you to list anything, no matter how impractical or outlandish it might seem at first. Then, go back and write notes about the possible obstacles, pros, or cons that you listed. Revisit Javier's example above if you get stuck. After you have written them all out, draw a star next to the ones that seem like the best action options. Try to come up with at least two or three, and reach out to others for help if you get stuck.

- _____
- _____
- _____
- _____
- _____
- _____
- _____
- _____
- _____

- _____
  - _____
- _____
  - _____
- _____
  - _____
- _____
  - _____

Whether you came up with one possible solution or ten, take some time to feel good about the work you're doing to improve your life. Now let's go to the last problem-solving step.

Select the Best Solution(s) and Take Action

You're doing great putting effort into these steps; the key for this section is to come up with plans to take action. If you're specific about the time line and steps you will take, you are more likely to follow through with them. Vague plans without concrete steps and time lines are less likely to be followed. It's also important to plan realistic steps for yourself and not overdo it. Be friendly to yourself as you come up with ways to change the situation. For example, this is what Javier came up with for his action plan:

1. Solution: Get a better-paying job.

   Action(s):

   - Spend the next two weeks updating my resume.

   - Spend at least a half hour on Saturdays looking for job openings in my field.

   - Apply to at least two jobs over the next two months.

2. Solution: Ask for a raise.

   Action(s):

   - During my annual review meeting next week, ask if it's possible to get a raise.

   - Plan out what I'm going to say and practice with one of my coworkers (Robert or Kenneth).

3.   Solution: Try to find a roommate.

     Action(s):

     •   Call Tiana today and ask her about her friend who was looking for a new roommate.

     •   If that doesn't work, try posting on social media to see if anyone else knows someone or try putting out an ad for a roommate.

4.   Solution: Cut back on expenses.

     Action(s):

     •   Reduce eating restaurant food from 5 times per week to 2 times per week by meal planning. I will start next Monday.

     •   Pay more attention to sales when buying clothes.

5.   Solution: Meet with a financial advisor.

     Action(s):

     •   I will look up my Employee Assistance Program tomorrow and schedule an appointment.

Step 3: Take Action

If you haven't yet, put a star next to the solutions that seem most practical and then plan how you will act on them, including specific tasks and time frames in the space below. The process of problem solving can help change some painful situations in your life.

1.   Solution: _____

     Action(s):

     •   _____

     •   _____

2.   Solution: _____

     Action(s):

     •   _____

     •   _____

3. Solution: _____

    Action(s):

    • _____

    • _____

4. Solution: _____

    Action(s):

    • _____

    • _____

5. Solution: _____

    Action(s):

    • _____

    • _____

I hope that reading Javier's example helped you learn about the process of problem solving. If it seems overwhelming, please know that it's not your fault. When you're suffering, it can be hard to see solutions. Take your time with it and give yourself credit for looking for ways to improve your life while you're feeling down. If you practice these three steps, you can learn to reduce the sting of some of life's stressors. I'm rooting for you!

How Can I Change My Perspective Through Cognitive-Behavioral Therapy?

Now that you have learned about problem solving, let's shift the focus to CBT strategies. It's a good time to revisit chapter 1 for the CBT model and the table of thinking errors before continuing this section.

Have you reviewed the model and thinking errors? Great! Let's look at how we can use this model to influence your thoughts, emotions, and behaviors. First, we'll identify your thoughts. Then we'll identify the type of thinking error that applies from the list in chapter 1. After the thinking patterns are identified, we'll work on creating a new, more helpful thought (called a "reframed thought").

CBT is different from positive thinking or trying to force yourself to be optimistic. The CBT process helps you notice inaccurate automatic thoughts and arrive at more accurate reframed thoughts that ring true. The purpose of identifying thinking patterns, examining evidence, and creating new thoughts is to reduce your emotional pain and clarify the situations you are in. If this feels like too much right now, I want to assure you that I'll help you through each step. As a therapist, I have worked with many struggling people who have learned CBT skills and watched their life improve as a result. Learning new skills is hard work, but I believe in you.

First, we'll work through an example by selecting two items from the list of Javier's sources of emotional pain. When you're thinking about items from your own list, try to select thoughts that have one or more of the thinking patterns highlighted in chapter 1. When describing your emotions, it helps to be specific. On the following page are some emotion words for you to choose from.

Emotion Words

Afraid	Discouraged	Hopeful	Panicked
Angry	Disgusted	Hopeless	Proud
Annoyed	Dread	Hurt	Regretful
Anxious	Embarrassed	Insecure	Resentful
Ashamed	Encouraged	Jealous	Sad
Bored	Excited	Joyful	Satisfied
Confused	Frustrated	Lonely	Scared
Content	Guilty	Nervous	Shocked
Curious	Happy	Neutral	Surprised
Disappointed	Helpless	Numb	Worried

Reframe Painful Thoughts (Javier's Example)

Thought: I'll be alone for the rest of my life.

Emotion(s): hopeless, dread, ashamed

Thinking error(s): emotional reasoning, fortune telling

Evidence for the thought: I feel that it's true, and I'm single right now.

Evidence against the thought: I can't tell the future. I have been in other relationships before this one. Other people get remarried after a divorce. There are opportunities for me to start dating again. I have family and friends who like to spend time with me.

New, reframed thought(s) in light of the evidence and without the thinking errors: It makes sense that I feel lonely right now after the divorce, but that doesn't mean I'll be alone for the rest of my life. I can't predict the future, and there are reasons to believe I might be in another relationship. Even if I'm not, that doesn't mean I'll be alone in my life. I have family and friends who love me.

Emotion(s): hopeful, relieved

Thought: All my friends think I'm a loser.

Emotion(s): embarrassed, hurt

Thinking error(s): labeling, mind reading, emotional reasoning

Evidence for the thought: I feel like they think that, but I don't really have any evidence.

Evidence against the thought: My friends tell me how much they love me. No one ever said I was a loser. If one of my friends was in my situation, I wouldn't think they were a loser.

New, reframed thought(s) in light of the evidence and without the thinking errors: It's understandable that I feel down right now after what I've been through, but I don't have any reason to believe my friends think I'm a loser. They are supportive of me and don't blame me for the divorce. Sometimes I feel like a loser because I miss Dan, but that doesn't mean anyone else feels that way or that it's true.

Emotions: calmer, reassured, less ashamed

As you can see from Javier's examples, CBT is focused on finding truth to reduce pain and suffering. Sometimes the people I work with in therapy say that they know the reframed thought is true, but it's hard to believe right away. If you feel that way, that is totally normal and expected. It takes practice and time to start embracing the new, more accurate thoughts. The key is to work through your thoughts, and when you notice yourself slipping into thinking errors, take time to remind yourself of the reframed thought. Act as if it is true, even if you don't feel it at first. With time, it will become easier to identify problematic thinking patterns and push back against them.

Now it's time to try the CBT framework with some of your own thoughts. The goal is to do the best that you can and practice the strategy. Be patient with yourself as you learn this new skill. If you get stuck, take a break and come back to it, and if you need extra help, ask a friend, therapist, or some other trusted person for help.

Reframe Painful Thoughts

Thought: _____

Emotion(s): _____

Thinking error(s): _____

Evidence for the thought: _____

_____

_____

Evidence against the thought: _____

_____

_____

New, reframed thought(s) in light of the evidence and without the thinking errors:

_____

_____

Emotion(s): _____

_____

How did that go? I hope you found it helpful! In therapy, I ask my patients to take pictures of their reframed thoughts with their phone—or print or write them out—so that they are easily accessed whenever the negative thoughts pop up. I suggest that you try that and see whether it works for you too. If it was hard to work through the exercise, that is okay. You'll get the hang of it. CBT might feel unnatural at first, because you are used to certain thinking patterns. But CBT is about changing those thinking patterns. With practice, it will start to feel more natural. Whenever you get stuck working through the above exercise, try asking yourself the questions below. Your responses will lead you to new ways to reframe your automatic thoughts.

- Am I seeing the situation as all bad because of one bad part?

- Are my expectations unrealistic or perfectionistic?

- Am I blaming myself for something I can't control?

- Am I assuming that one bad event means I'm doomed to a bad life?

- Am I missing something positive about the situation?

- Am I viewing negative comments as truer than positive comments?

- Am I considering anything less than perfect to be worthless?

- Am I guessing what other people think of me?

- Am I guessing other people's intentions?

- Am I predicting the future without really knowing what will happen?

- Am I overestimating the likelihood of something bad happening?

- Am I underestimating my ability to cope with hard situations?

- Am I labeling myself or others?

- Is there another possible explanation for the situation?

The Pain of Feeling Like a Burden

Before we conclude this chapter, I want to make a special note of a feeling that is common among people who have suicidal thoughts. Research shows that many people who want to kill themselves view themselves as a burden on others (Chu et al., 2017). Is this true for you? Do you feel like the people in your life would be better off if you were gone? If you feel this way, it must hurt so much to feel that your loved ones would be better off without you. I want you to know that you're not alone in those feelings and that your loved ones are *not* better off without you.

Sometimes it's hard to see this truth in our own lives and easier to see it when we look at a situation outside of our own. For example, Nirvana singer Kurt Cobain wrote in his suicide note, "Please keep going Courtney [his wife], for Frances [their daughter]. For her life, which will be so much happier without me." Kurt's words are tragic, because he felt that his wife and daughter would be better off without him. The second tragedy is that he was mistaken. Frances was two years old then and is now in her twenties. She's spoken about the pain of never getting to know her dad, despite his belief that her life would be better without him in it. Courtney Love, his widow, has also said how hurt she felt after he died and that she still misses him to this day. Like every person, Kurt was imperfect and had parts of him that were hard for his family, but they still wanted him to stay with them and be in their lives. He was valued by his family, friends, and many other people.

Struggling does not make you unlovable or unworthy of a good life. When you're in a low place, you may feel like someone who brings others down. It's not your fault that you feel that way, but you do have the ability to push back on those thoughts through the CBT strategies mentioned above. If you're feeling like a burden, try the following:

- *Check your thinking patterns.* Are you jumping to conclusions, discounting the positive, or having emotional reasoning that tricks you into thinking your friends and family would be better off without you? If so, try working through the CBT worksheet to come up with a more accurate, compassionate reframed thought.

- *Check the evidence.* Is there evidence that people appreciate, like, or love having you in their life? If you're having trouble finding the evidence on your own, ask trusted people in your life how you positively contribute to theirs. When they respond, write down what they say and remind yourself of it whenever those feelings of being a burden creep in.

- *Take action.* Sometimes, it's easier to influence intense feelings about yourself by changing your actions instead of wrestling with your thoughts. Try finding ways to contribute (e.g., say something nice to someone, offer to help out, volunteer, listen to someone) and give yourself credit for those actions as powerful proof that people are better off with you here and in their lives. If that doesn't fit for you right now, try spending time with people who love and appreciate you. Being around people who express their love for you can ease the intensity of feeling like a burden.

It doesn't take grand contributions for people to want you in their lives. You being you is enough.

Summary of Key Points

- People have suicidal thoughts because they want to escape emotional pain that feels unbearable.

- You can reduce the intensity of the emotional pain by changing the situation (through problem solving), changing your perspective (through CBT), or both.

- If you're feeling like a burden, try working through those thoughts with CBT or by taking actions to reduce that feeling.

Reflection

What thoughts, ideas, and feelings did you have while reading and working through this chapter? Were there certain parts you didn't relate to? What parts did you relate to most? What did you learn?

CHAPTER 6

Foster Self-Compassion and Acceptance

If you tried problem solving and CBT strategies to ease your pain and you're still hurting, that doesn't mean something is wrong with you or that you're to blame. It just means that different kinds of coping skills are needed right now. You might be in difficult circumstances that you can't change—or at least can't change quickly (e.g., toxic work environment, caring for a sick loved one, a natural disaster). Some pain is unavoidable even when we try to solve our problems and shift our perspectives.

In the last chapter, we learned that Javier experienced the heartbreak of missing Dan after their divorce. That part of Javier's pain did not involve the kind of thinking errors that CBT addresses. He tried problem solving through couples therapy, but that did not prevent the divorce and sadness that followed. This is an example of the type of situation where Javier could soothe his pain by being compassionate toward himself and his emotional experiences rather than fighting them. In this chapter, you'll learn how to (1) increase awareness of your inner experiences through mindfulness, (2) foster self-compassion, and (3) cultivate acceptance.

Increase Awareness

How often are you truly in the moment? Do you tend to have a lot going on in the back of your mind: a running to-do list, a replay of past conversations, and worries about the future? If so, you are like most people who are not totally focused on the present. Our brains naturally latch on to different things throughout the day. That can make it hard to notice how we're relating to ourselves and our emotions. The exercises below will help you strengthen your observational skills so that you notice how you're treating yourself and how you're feeling. Increased awareness of your thoughts, emotions, and behaviors help you find the coping skills that best fit the situation.

Awareness of Experiences

Let's start this exercise by setting a timer for five minutes. After you set the timer, use the space below to write down thoughts, emotions, physical sensations, and other things you notice. Are you feeling calm, nervous, or another emotion? What sounds do you hear? What colors do you see? Are your muscles tense or relaxed? The goal is to simply notice some of your experiences.

- _____
- _____
- _____
- _____
- _____
- _____
- _____
- _____
- _____

Did you finish the exercise? Excellent job! How did you feel while creating the list? Was it easy or hard to stay focused? However you felt, I want to assure you that it is okay. The point of the exercise is to increase attention toward your thoughts and feelings, and I'm sure that happened as you participated. That means you're already practicing a skill for observing your experiences called mindfulness. Nice work!

Increase Mindfulness

Thich Nhat Hanh (1976) described mindfulness as a way to observe your inner experiences and surroundings without judgment. When you have pain in your life that you want to address, mindfulness is a tool that you can use to find the space to process it. Mindfulness can be challenging at first, especially if you're used to pushing away unwanted feelings. With repeated practice, you can strengthen your mindfulness skills. For the purposes of this workbook, the goal of mindfulness is to build awareness of your inner experiences, not to completely empty your mind of all thoughts. Mindfulness is also useful for grounding yourself in moments when you feel disconnected or preoccupied.

If you're interested in reading more on this topic, Thich Nhat Hanh's *Miracle of Mindfulness* has a number of mindfulness exercises in it. Below I have listed exercises that I've found especially helpful as a therapist and in my own life. I recommend giving them each a try to build your mindfulness skills. After you have tried them all, you can pick the ones you like best for future use.

Mindfulness Practice

- *Focus on your breath:* Breathe in and out. Don't try to change the pace of your breath. Just notice it. When thoughts enter your mind—and they will—notice them and refocus on your breath as soon as you can. You can practice this by setting a goal (e.g., for ten breaths or two minutes). This is hard at first, but it will get easier with repeated tries. A benefit of learning to be mindful through a breathing focus is that it's something always available to you in a variety of situations.

- *Focus on music:* Some people find mindfulness of their breath hard because of the quiet. Mindfulness to music is another great option. I recommend selecting a song of any genre without lyrics. As you listen, notice the different instruments or when the melody or volume changes. Notice any feelings or thoughts that arise and then bring your mind back to the music.

- *Focus on eating:* There is a classic mindfulness exercise that involves raisins. While this works well, I prefer to practice with candy. You can select any food that you like. Once you have selected the food, put it in your hand and look at it. See what you notice about the food that you have missed in past experiences when you weren't paying close attention. How does the light reflect on it? Is it all one color or different colors? Once you have spent some time looking at it, put a piece into your mouth without chewing. What is the texture? Is it soft, smooth, or rough? Notice the urge to chew or swallow and wait a bit before acting on it. When you're ready, bite into it. Notice the flavor. Does it change the longer you chew? What else do you notice?

- *Focus on showering:* This has been a favorite practice of many of my therapy patients, because it's a convenient way to incorporate mindfulness into their daily routines. When you shower, focus on the feeling of the water. What is the temperature? How is the pressure? Notice as steam starts to fill the room. As you go through your washing routine, notice the scent, texture, and other aspects of the soap, shampoo, and washcloth. As thoughts come into your mind, refocus on the process of showering.

- *Focus on creating:* Some people feel most aware when they are engaged in some type of creative activity. Common activities that can be useful for mindfulness practice include cooking, coloring, playing an instrument, and painting. Try these activities while focusing on the individual steps of the process. When your mind strays from the task at hand, practice pulling your attention back to the activity.

Some people find mindfulness relaxing, but don't fret if you don't. Mindfulness exercises are different from relaxation exercises because the goal is to increase your awareness rather than change your experience. As an observer of your thoughts and feelings, you can create space to relate to yourself and your inner experiences differently than you have in the past. When you step back from your experiences as an observer, it allows you to have more influence over how you relate to them.

Increase Self-Compassion

Using your mindfulness skills, pay attention to the self-talk you are doing right now. What do you notice about how you speak to yourself and what you think about yourself? In my work as a therapist, I meet people who are incredibly kind and loving to others but offer no grace to themselves. Is that also true of you? If it is, do you think your self-criticism is connected to any of these kinds of experiences?

- growing up with a parent, grandparent, or other person who harshly criticized you

- being in an abusive or otherwise toxic relationship

- spending time in an environment where you were treated as unworthy

- holding perfectionistic standards and berating yourself if you fall short

- being targeted with discrimination, harassment, or bullying

- working in a high-pressure setting where mistakes are not tolerated

- just the way you've always felt

If it was something else, write what it is in the space below.

_____

_____

_____

Regardless of where your self-criticism comes from, with practice, you can approach yourself with more kindness. To be clear, self-compassion doesn't mean that you stop striving for change or improvement. It means that you are encouraging and understanding of yourself as you work toward goals rather than demeaning and cruel. Psychological scientist Kristin Neff (2003) defines self-compassion as "a way of relating to ourselves in times of suffering that is characterized by increased kindness and reduced self-judgment." I share this definition because some people are afraid that they'll lose their ambition if they start being nicer to themselves. I have never seen this happen in many years of therapy practice.

Please take a moment to think of something stressful that happened in the past few weeks. How did you relate to yourself when it was happening? Did you compare yourself to others, telling yourself that they would have handled it better? Were you ashamed for feeling the way that you did? If you responded to yourself in a critical manner, what happened to your feelings? Usually, people's stress gets worse when they're self-critical, because the shame adds another layer to their suffering. In addition to feeling bad, these reactions are unhelpful. They often lead to lower motivation due to a lack of confidence and unhealthy coping strategies (e.g., avoidance). For those reasons, self-compassion is not just about "being nice" to yourself. It's about being honest with yourself in a way that maximizes the chances of choosing a healthy path forward.

Research shows that self-compassion is linked to good mental health (Bluth and Neff, 2018). The exercise below includes several strategies to help you learn to relate to yourself in a kinder manner. I have been amazed by the transformative power of self-compassion in many of my patients' lives, and I hope that you experience that too.

Self-Compassion Practice

- *Imagine someone comforting you:* Think of a friend or family member who has helped you before in times of trouble. Have you identified that person? Great! Now imagine that person is sitting next to you. What would they do to comfort you? Give you a hug? Tell you it's not your fault? Would they say they know it's hard and remind you that you don't have to go through it alone? Would they sympathize and say they're sorry that you're going through this? Try to vividly imagine the person saying these things to you. It can be tough to make these compassionate words and gestures toward yourself, but it is often easier to imagine someone else talking to you in this manner.

- *Imagine a friend or loved one in the same situation as you:* What would you say to comfort them? What would you do to show that you support them? Try writing a letter to them with words of support. Now read that letter aloud to yourself and see how it makes you feel. Did it lessen your suffering? I hope that it did.

- *Draw a picture of yourself as viewed by someone who loves you:* What positive qualities do they see in you? How is their love expressed when they see you? Try drawing a picture of yourself surrounded by symbols of love and compassion (e.g., nature scenes, a heart, two hands clasping, people hugging, spiritual symbols). The quality of the drawing is not important. The idea is to find different ways to relate to yourself. Sometimes artistic expression can shift you toward greater self-compassion when you otherwise feel stuck in your head.

- *Say self-compassionate statements to yourself aloud:* Sometimes hearing the words can help them sink in. If you're feeling stuck, here are some sample phrases to say to yourself (pick the ones that most apply), plus space at the bottom where you can add your own:

  - I am doing the best I can.

  - I am worthy of love and care even when I feel down.

  - This is not my fault.

- I did the best I could with the information that I had at the time. Nobody's perfect.

- My feelings and experiences are valid even if other people don't see things the same way.

- It's understandable that I'm in pain right now. It's okay to feel.

- _____

- _____

- _____

- _____

- _____

- *Try self-compassion with touch and physical comfort:* Here are some ideas for this exercise: gently hold your hands together, take a shower or bubble bath, stroke your pet's fur, hug a loved one, put on your most comfortable clothes, or wrap yourself in your favorite blanket. Try viewing yourself and your body as worthy of care and kindness instead of criticism and cruelty.

- *Look up Virginia Satir's prose poem "My Declaration of Self-Esteem" on the internet:* Practice reading it aloud every day for a week. See if it makes a difference in how you see yourself.

Think about how you can keep working on those self-compassionate statements. Will you say them every morning or every night? Will you put them in your calendar on your phone, so they pop up once a day? You can also print them or draw them and post them in places in your home where you will see them regularly. Find a way that works for you to build this practice of self-compassion. Cultivating self-compassion is a journey that takes repeated practice in difficult moments. It can feel strange to start relating to yourself with more kindness if you're used to putting yourself down. It will probably start to feel more natural over time. You are worthy of compassion. I know you can do it!

The Benefits of Accepting Unwanted Emotions and Situations

"Our current mental-hygiene philosophy stresses the idea that people ought to be happy, that unhappiness is a symptom of maladjustment. Such a value system might be responsible for the fact that the burden of unavoidable unhappiness is increased by the unhappiness about being unhappy." —Dr. Edith Weisskopf-Joelson (1955)

The above quote captures something I have seen time after time among my therapy patients. They'll experience a hardship in their life and feel unhappy about it. Then, rather than viewing their unhappiness as a perfectly natural response to a stressful situation, they view it as a personal flaw that should be fixed. The message that you should be happy—and if you're not, you're doing something wrong—can be sent within cultures, workplaces, and other environments. Some send the message that you are completely responsible for your own happiness and have failed if you haven't figured out how to be happy.

I see this a lot in therapy surrounding grief, the end of romantic relationships, missed opportunities, and the end of friendships. There's an idea that there is a time line you should follow—a period when you can feel bad and a time when you should move on. If you haven't moved on, people start suggesting that you just stop thinking about it or try harder to think positively. Have you ever experienced something like this? Perhaps you're in pain and then the pain becomes worse because you try to stop being in pain, which adds more pain about your inability to let go of the pain. What a vicious cycle!

When you're stuck in a situation that you cannot control and you're trying to be happy, it makes sense to try to deny that it's happening. You might replay situations from the past over and over in your mind and think about how you could have prevented them. When reality is hard to face, it's natural to try these avoidance and denial strategies. Paradoxically, the struggle to push reality away can make your suffering grow. When you replay the past in your mind, trying to imagine it going differently than it did, you might temporarily feel more control over the situation. However, over the long term, it makes the painful emotions come back stronger, accompanied by additional self-blame. Again, this is all completely understandable. Painful emotions motivate us to turn away or imagine situations where they aren't happening. And this is especially true if you are experiencing pressure to be happy from your environment. Please approach yourself with compassion if you notice those patterns in yourself as you start to reflect on those experiences below.

When you think back on your life, what are things that happened to you that felt especially unfair? As a therapist, I have seen patients who experienced extremely painful situations, such as the loss of a child or a parent, infertility, or a tragic accident. In their pain, they desperately search for explanations and sometimes land on self-blame or a belief that they're being punished. Humans are driven to make sense of the world, even the hardest parts of it. The attempt to find meaning in a tragic situation is nothing to feel ashamed of, but it can lead to feeling stuck. Family therapist Virginia Satir said, "Life is not what it's supposed to be. It's what it is. The way you cope with it is what makes the difference." Let's consider the following situation as an example.

> When Christine was getting a physical, her doctor expressed concerns about abnormal lab results and low body weight. Christine knew she focused on food and exercising a lot, but she didn't realize it was negatively affecting her health. The doctor referred her to get evaluated for an eating disorder, and the therapist formally diagnosed her with one. Christine felt numb as she left the therapist's office and got into her car. She started the car, and as she was driving, a wave of shame washed over her. Christine felt embarrassed that her eating habits had gotten so out of hand. In the past, she had always worked so hard to be healthy. The idea of being treated for an eating disorder and having to tell her loved ones felt scary. She started sobbing, overwhelmed with feelings of helplessness and self-blame.

It's makes sense that Christine is experiencing all of these intense emotions. Once they settle down a bit, she'll have to decide what she's going to do about it. She has some different options:

- *Denial:* Christine could continue her current eating patterns and try to convince herself that the doctor and therapist are wrong. She could decide to avoid her feelings through starvation, alcohol, or substance use and tell herself she doesn't need help. The downsides to this approach are that she will continue suffering from the negative effects, including damage to her body, which may lead to even greater pain in her future.

- *Self-blame, self-criticism:* Christine could tell herself that she should have prevented the situation and never let it spiral out of control. She could decide that she is to blame for the eating disorder and that it's her responsibility to snap out of it on her own. The downside of this path is that she would also experience sadness and shame related to feeling terrible about who she is and the situation she is in on top of struggling with an eating disorder.

- *Self-compassion, acceptance:* Christine could approach herself in a friendly, loving manner while recognizing that she has a serious issue that needs to be addressed. She could accept the reality of the situation without blaming herself and acknowledge that she needs help. The upside to this is that Christine can work to effectively reduce a source of pain while being kind to herself. This approach allows her to hold space for her feelings while encouraging herself to face reality and her need for treatment.

As you can see, if Christine accepts her situation, she has the best chance to get well and reduce her long-term suffering. It's often easier for us to see that from the outside than within our own lives. The truth is that acceptance of the past and present can relieve the additional hurt and frustration that comes with denying painful realities. It's important to remember that acceptance does not mean that you approve of the situation you're in. It doesn't mean that you don't want to make changes in the future. It simply means that you are taking an effective approach to a situation you cannot change, or as Carl Rogers said, "The curious paradox is that when I accept myself just as I am, then I can change."

Increase Acceptance

Using your mindfulness skills, what feelings and thoughts did you notice as you read the previous section? What would you like to accept in your own life? Please take out your journal and write a list. Please note that acceptance can focus only on the past or present, because we don't yet know what the future will bring. What did you select? Is it something about yourself or another person? Is it about a regret that you have? Is it a circumstance that you are currently in? Take your time. I know you can do this.

Now that you have picked something you want to accept, let's talk about how you can cultivate acceptance. People work toward acceptance through all kinds of pathways. Sometimes we build acceptance through experiences with other people. When I was in school, I told a friend that I felt bad that I wasn't as energetic as another student we knew. Later in my career, I had a similar conversation with another friend about feeling inferior to a peer who was more active than me. Both times, my friends looked at me and said something to the effect of, "Well, what if you're the kind of person who just needs to take breaks and rest more?" It seems simple, but it had honestly never occurred to me to just be okay with being different. When I'm struggling with acceptance in that area, I replay those conversations in my mind. Do you have any experiences like that in your life that you could revisit to nurture acceptance? I recommend taking some time to think about them or to write about them in your journal.

This workbook is focused on finding the tools that best fit your life. I thank you for keeping an open mind and having the willingness to try different approaches. Another acceptance strategy is to picture what you might feel like if you accepted yourself or the situation. Imagining it or acting as if you accept the situation might bring you a step closer to experiencing it. Remember, you get to choose what you want to accept. You do not need to apply this skill to any situations where it is unhelpful to you.

Acceptance Practice

Find a quiet space to relax and imagine how it would feel to accept yourself. If you notice yourself wanting to turn away from acceptance, gently bring yourself back into focus by reading the statements or trying some of the suggestions below.

- My situation is painful right now. I can't change the past, but I can try to accept it.

- Acceptance does not mean that I like how my life is right now. It means that I'm acknowledging it instead of trying to avoid it.

- I accept all my feelings, emotions, and thoughts right now. There is nothing wrong with me for feeling my emotions.

- Replaying past events does not change them. This is where I am right now, and I can accept it as reality, even if I don't like it.

- Right now, in this moment, I accept my reality. Every part of it. I'm taking a break from trying to push it away or control it.

Some people find it helpful to pray or read pieces of scripture to increase acceptance. For example, some of my patients have found the Serenity Prayer useful, which you can find on the internet. Others find it helpful to look for phrases, poems, or lyrics that encourage acceptance (e.g., "Let It Be" by the Beatles). What actions might you take if you truly accepted yourself or the situation? Try taking those actions and see if that builds acceptance. Are there other ways to increase acceptance? Explore your ideas in the space below.

_____

_____

_____

_____

_____

Summary of Key Points

- When problem solving or CBT skills don't help with the pain you're experiencing, you can try mindfulness, self-compassion, and acceptance exercises.

- Mindfulness skills increase awareness about how you relate to yourself and your situation. Repeated practice strengthens the skill.

- As you work on making changes, try to relate to yourself in a kind, friendly manner. Acceptance reduces suffering and self-blame.

Reflection

What thoughts, ideas, and feelings did you have while reading and working through this chapter? Were there certain parts you didn't relate to? What parts did you relate to most? What did you learn?

CHAPTER 7

Increase Hope

When you're in pain, it's perfectly natural to want to make that pain go away. If your pain is severe or long-lasting, you may be thinking, *I'll feel this bad forever,* or *Nothing will ever change for me.* Beliefs that you're doomed to a horrible future lead to feeling helpless, and suicide may start to seem like the only way to escape your misery. If you're experiencing painful life circumstances, I want you to know that your desire to hurt less is completely valid. It's also important to know that, even in the face of extreme hardships, there are reasons to hold on.

Build Hope

When you're feeling suicidal, it's hard to find hope without guidance. It can feel like you're stuck in a dark place without a single spark of light. This chapter focuses on creating sparks of light. The exercises don't attempt to instill hope through shallow, superficial, or clichéd ways. Instead, we'll work together to find reasons for hope using strategies from therapy and psychological research.

The exercises are designed with different kinds of situations in mind. You'll find that some are more relevant to your life than others. I recommend reading through all of them and then focusing on the ones that work best for you right now. Some of the suggested activities take less effort, while others take more in-depth work. Use the ones that fit best with your current mind state and energy level.

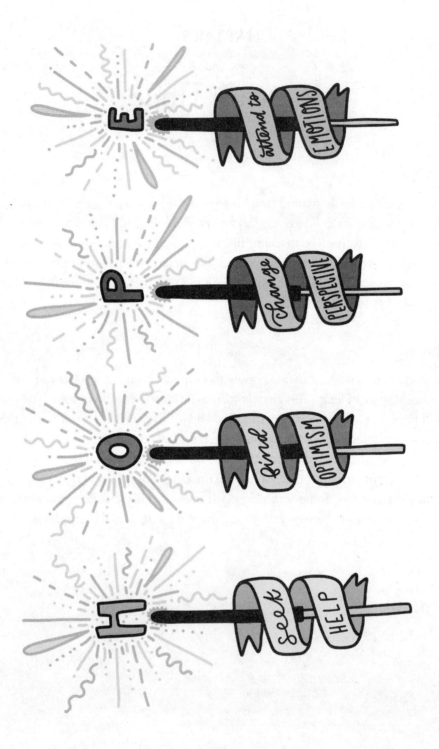

Illustration by Alyse Ruriani

Each letter of the acronym on the previous page represents a hope-building strategy. It was designed so that you can cut out the page and put it up somewhere—or you can take a picture of it with your phone, so you can look at it any time you need a reminder. You can personalize it by coloring it, adding pictures, or doing anything else that feels right to you. The chapter is split into four sections, one for each letter in the acronym: seek Help, find Optimism, change Perspective, and attend to Emotions. When you feel hopeless, it can be hard to think about trying these out. Special care was taken so that the exercises walk you through small, manageable steps.

Seek Help

If you're considering suicide, you may feel like a burden on others or like you're all alone in the world (Van Orden et al., 2010). Understandably, these kinds of beliefs make it hard to ask for help. It's tragic that breaking out of isolation can be the toughest at the exact time you need people the most. I start this chapter with this step—seek help—toward building hope because reaching out to others is one of the most powerful methods for feeling better. Support from others can reduce pain, shame, and loneliness.

Overcome Obstacles

Common help-seeking obstacles are listed below. Mark the ones you most relate to with an *X*. For each one you have marked with an *X*, read the passage below it for suggestions on working through that obstacle.

_____   I am all alone in this. There is no one I can turn to.

Are you unintentionally crossing off options for people you could turn to for help? Gently encourage yourself to brainstorm about all the possible people available, including those you might have prematurely ruled out. These could include a friend, family member, coworker, neighbor, clergy member, physician, therapist, peer mental health support person, suicide hotline, or local mental health group. If finances are a barrier to working with a therapist, there may be affordable or free options available near you (e.g., a university psychology training clinic, therapists with a sliding scale fee). You can usually find out about these options by calling a local mental health hotline for referrals. Most therapists who have a sliding scale fee will put that information on their website. In addition, mental health support groups and social groups situated within houses of worship or community centers are sometimes free or low cost.

_____   I should be able to fix this myself.

The most effective way for you to fix this yourself is to use the resources available to you, which means letting go of the idea that people overcome serious issues on their own. Instead, focus on accepting the reality that people need others to get through hardships. Human beings are built to lean on each other in times of need. None of us can work through all of our problems alone. We all need help at times.

_____   If I ask for help, that means I'm weak.

This statement is the exact opposite of the truth. Asking for help is hard, and it requires a lot of strength. It's a myth that suicide is related to weakness. Exceptionally strong, tough people are afflicted by the pain of suicidal thoughts. Many find their way through their hardships with the grace of others' assistance. Imagine a close friend or family member in the same situation as you. Would you view them as weak for seeking help? Try to foster the same compassion for yourself that you would have for your loved ones.

_____   If I tell people about my problems, I will burden them. Or if people knew how I really felt, they wouldn't like me.

People who lose a friend or family member to suicide often wish they had known how much their loved one was hurting. People grieving after losing someone often say they would have done anything in their power to help. They sometimes say that some of the pain of their loss is specifically because they had not been able to provide support, because they did not know. You may be thinking that applies to most people, but you're an exception to this rule. I promise that many people experiencing suicidal thoughts feel that way too. You are worthy of receiving love and help from people. Please give it a try. If you've tried reaching out and find that people don't know how to support you, consider sharing appendix A with them.

_____   Even if I reach out, nothing will help me feel better.

I can understand why you feel this way when you're at a low point, especially if you've had negative experiences in the past, but please know that there are ways to make life feel better. The evidence is available in scientific research and in the many personal stories of people paving paths to joy and purpose. It's natural to feel skeptical of the idea that your life could improve when you've been struggling. Fortunately, you don't have to let go of that skepticism to give these exercises a try. You can approach them with an open mind in the presence of doubt. The fact that you're reading this workbook means you're already doing this and deserve credit for taking these important steps.

_____   I don't know how to ask for help.

Sometimes it's hard to find the words to tell someone you're struggling. Here are some suggestions for starting the conversation:

- "I have been feeling down lately. Can we talk about it?"

- "I have been really unhappy, and I'm not sure how to make things better. Would you mind helping me think through it?"

- "I'm afraid to open up about this, but I'm having a hard time and would like to talk to someone about it."

The next step is to commit to your help-seeking plan by listing people or groups to contact for help in the exercise below. The more realistic and practical your choices are, the more likely you will be to follow through with them. Review the above section, as needed, to overcome any hurdles that come up. You can do this! (A copy of this worksheet is available on the New Harbinger website for downloading and printing: http://www.newharbinger.com/47025.)

Help-Seeking Plan

- Name of person or organization: _____

  How I will contact them (e.g., text, in person, phone, email):

  _____

  When I will contact them (day, time):

  _____

  The kind of help I'll ask for:

  _____

- Name of person or organization: _____

  How I will contact them (e.g., text, in person, phone, email):

  _____

  When I will contact them (day, time):

  _____

  The kind of help I'll ask for:

  _____

- Name of person or organization: _____

  How I will contact them (e.g., text, in person, phone, email):

  _____

  When I will contact them (day, time):

  _____

  The kind of help I'll ask for:

  _____

Sometimes people in our lives—even people we have never met—can help us find hope. Are there actors, musicians, athletes, writers, or other people who inspire you?

Find Inspiration from Others

Below, write the names of people who inspire you. Look up pictures or articles about them. You can save pictures or quotes by them on your phone or print them out so that you can look at them whenever you need a boost of hope.

- _____

- _____

- _____

- _____

- _____

Find Reasons for Optimism

In this section—the O of HOPE—we focus on optimism. When you're feeling suicidal, a type of tunnel vision can take over that makes it hard to see future bright spots. This section provides tools to help you find those sparks of light.

Look Forward to Things

In the space below, list any upcoming event, big or small, that you expect to feel good. What do you look forward to? What would you hate to miss out on? This exercise chips away at that foundation of hopelessness that says you'll feel bad forever. Some examples have been provided to get you started.

Example:

- finding out if my team will win the championship this year

- that new movie that I really want to see

- seeing my niece graduate from high school

- seeing the leaves change color in the fall

- a cup of coffee from my favorite coffee shop in the morning

- finding out what happens at the end of the book I'm reading

- gardening next summer

- sunsets

- going to my cousin's wedding

- traveling

Your list:

- _____

- _____

- _____

- _____

- _____

- _____

- _____

- _____

- _____

At age forty-five, Stephen had a family to support, including a child with diabetes, so a steady income and quality health insurance were of prime importance to him. When he was laid off from his job, Stephen began thinking, I can't handle this. I'm not going to get through this. He saw no way out of his circumstances and felt ashamed for not being able to provide for his family. Stephen started thinking his family would be better off without him. In those dire circumstances, Stephen considered killing himself.

Like Stephen, many people who feel suicidal have a hard time seeing the strengths and abilities that they have to skillfully navigate situations. You may feel that you're unable to cope with the challenges ahead. The exercise below is an opportunity to find evidence from your own life that can help you believe this statement: "Life is very hard now, but I am capable of coping with it."

Build Confidence Through Past Experiences

- What is a challenge that you have faced in the past that you didn't think you would be able to get through (e.g., a romantic breakup, a job loss, depression, financial struggles, medical issues, or another life stressor)?

  _____

  _____

  _____

- How did you get through that difficult time? List the strengths, skills, and resources you used to get through that situation (e.g., relying on friends, maintaining a sense of humor, problem solving).

  - _____

  - _____

  - _____

  - _____

  - _____

  - _____

  - _____

- Considering the evidence in that list, what can you say to yourself to get through what you're struggling with right now? Sample self-statements have been listed to get you started. Please add your own at the bottom.

  - I'm strong enough to survive hard times.

  - I have skills to cope with life's challenges.

  - I have made it through tough times before, and I can do it again.

  - It may feel impossible now, but I can make it through this.

  - _____

  - _____

  - _____

  - _____

More Reasons for Optimism

Building on the previous exercises in this section, list some additional reasons for optimism about the future. Some examples have been given to get you started.

- There are good people in my life and the world who can help me [name them]:

  _____

- My life has been good before, and it can be again.

- I can't predict the future. Things could change for the better. If I kill myself I'll never find out.

- People suffering as badly or worse than I am have gone on to feel better and live meaningful lives [name them]:

  _____

- There are resources out there (e.g., therapy, financial assistance) that can help me improve my life:

  _____

  _____

  _____

  _____

  _____

Change Perspective

In this section we move on to the P of HOPE—perspective. Why do some people become hopeless in the face of stressors while others do not? Some factors include life circumstances (e.g., access to financial and other resources), personality differences, and surrounding environments. One scientific theory proposes that hope levels are influenced by people's beliefs about what negative life events mean about them and their lives (Abramson et al., 1989; Liu et al., 2015). Specifically, people become hopeless when they attribute stressors to internal (themselves), global (related to all situations of that type), and stable (unchanging) factors. For example, consider these three different reactions to the end of a romantic relationship.

Alex broke off a relationship with his girlfriend, Olivia, after three years. Olivia felt that it came out of nowhere. Alex explained that he was no longer in love with Olivia, even though he still wanted to be friends.

Scenario 1: Olivia feels sad that her relationship with Alex ended. She can't stop thinking about how she should have done things differently so that he would still want to be with her (internal attribution). Olivia valued Alex's opinion and felt that his rejection meant that she was not a good enough person for him or anyone else (global attribution). She took the relationship's end as meaning that she's inherently unlovable and would be alone forever (stable attribution).

Scenario 2: Olivia feels sad that her relationship with Alex ended. She can't stop thinking about how it is all Alex's fault (external attribution). Olivia felt that this situation was relevant to their relationship but nothing else about her or her life (specific attribution). She took the relationship's end to mean that she would be single now but would likely find someone else to date in the future (unstable attribution).

Scenario 3: Olivia feels sad that her relationship with Alex ended. She understands that she made some mistakes in the relationship—like all people do—but that it doesn't necessarily mean something is wrong with her as a person (mixed internal and external attribution). Olivia plans on taking some time to reflect on her patterns in romantic relationships to see if there are ways to improve, but she thinks other romantic relationships could work better than her one with Alex (specific attribution). She plans to take time to heal from the breakup and feels optimistic that she'll find another partner in the future (unstable attribution).

Shift Your Viewpoint

As you can see above, the same stressful life event impacted Olivia differently depending on what it meant to her in each scenario. People don't purposely view stressors in hopeless ways, but they can give stable or internal attributions to these events automatically when they're struggling with depression or other types of mental health issues. The good news is that, once you're aware of these attributions and how they affect your viewpoint, you can learn to push back on them. The worksheet below guides you through a process of seeing your situation through new perspectives. Sometimes people think that this kind of process means you're "just thinking positive" or "lying to yourself." However, the key with this next exercise is that, just like CBT in chapter 5, you're working to make your interpretations more accurate by looking at evidence you may have missed in your first response to the situation.

Internal   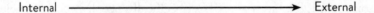   External

Internal attributions include thoughts such as *It is all my fault*. The exercise below will help you think through external factors too. The goal is to see whether *It is partially my fault* or *It is not my fault* is truer and therefore more hopeful.

1.   What is a current stressful situation that you are in?

_____

2. What percentage (out of 100) do you blame yourself for the situation and why?

   • The situation is _____ percent my fault.

   • It is [circle one: **completely, somewhat, not at all**] my fault because [write more detail in the space below]:

   _____

   _____

3. Are there any outside factors in the situation that were not in your control? Feel free to ask others for help identifying them and then list them below.

   _____

   _____

4. If you have considered external factors and still feel you are completely to blame, is there a way to give yourself some compassion? Were you doing the best you knew how to at the time? If a friend was in the same situation as you, would you put all the blame on them? Why or why not? Are you applying harsher standards to yourself than you would to other people? Try to be fair to yourself as you evaluate your role in the situation.

   _____

   _____

5. After considering the information you wrote about above, please answer these questions again while considering what you learned above.

   • The situation is _____ percent my fault.

   • It is [circle one: **totally, somewhat, not at all**] my fault because (write more detail in the space below):

   _____

   _____

Global ——————————————————→ Specific

Global attributions include beliefs like *This situation means something about my overall worth as a person*, or *Because someone treated me poorly in this situation, all other relationships will be affected*. The exercise below will help you think about whether your beliefs are overgeneralizing. The goal is to see whether statements such as

This conversation didn't work out well, but that doesn't mean I am incapable of communicating effectively or *This one situation didn't work out, but it doesn't mean that nothing else will work out for me* would be more accurate, hopeful interpretations.

- What does this situation mean about you as a person?

  _____

  _____

- What does it mean about other situations in your life?

  _____

  _____

- Consider the questions below to see whether you can make your attributions more specific and less global.

  - Have you been in similar situations (e.g., related to work, friendships, relationships, etc.) where you had a better outcome? List those other situations.

    _____

    _____

  - Are you overly focused on negative experiences and ignoring the positive ones? Name some of the positive counterexamples that come to mind.

    _____

    _____

  - What areas of your life will not be affected by this stressful situation?

    _____

    _____

  - If the stressor is affecting other areas of your life, are there ways to minimize its impact? Are there things you can do to prevent it from spilling into other areas?

    _____

    _____

In light of what you wrote about above, answer the questions from the beginning of this exercise again. Hopefully, your perspective has shifted, such that your interpretations are more specific (to this situation) and less global (having significance about you as a person or your life overall).

- What does this situation mean about you as a person?

_____

- What does it mean about other situations in your life?

_____

Stable ——————————————→ Unstable

Stable attributions such as *Things will never get better* and *Nothing will ever change for me* are closely linked to hopelessness about having a better life in the future. Use the exercise below to examine evidence that moves your interpretation of the stressor from stable to changeable. The goal is to evaluate whether beliefs such as *Things are bad now, but they might get better* or *My life might improve* better fit the facts.

- What is the characteristic about yourself or your situation that you think will never change?

_____

_____

- It might feel like things will always be this way, but can you name some situations where it was different in the past?

_____

_____

- Are there tools you can use to influence the course of the future? Are there ways to work on yourself or change your situation that increase the chances for future change?

_____

_____

- If you and the situation truly won't change, is it possible that the way you feel about it could change? For example, are there people in situations like yours who have a different outlook? Have you had a useful change of perspective on a painful situation before?

_____

_____

After working through the questions above, do you see your situation differently? I suggest writing in your journal about how your perspective has changed and why.

Attend to Emotions

This is the final section of HOPE, the *E*—emotions. Your painful emotions may be communicating a need to you. In this section, we'll explore your feelings and try to see what kind of response might be most helpful for softening the pain.

Respond to Feelings

1. How are you feeling right now? Revisit the list of emotion words in chapter 5 if needed.

    _____

2. What prompted those emotions? If you're not sure, that's okay.

    _____

3. Please take a moment to validate your feelings by telling yourself the following:

    My feelings are valid. Emotional pain is not a sign that I am flawed or weak. It is a sign that something hurts and that I need additional care.

4. Sometimes attending to your emotions simply means acknowledging your feelings and telling yourself that it is okay to feel how you feel. Other times, it means taking further action to change the situation that is causing pain. What can you do to attend to your emotions right now? If you're not sure, review exercises in chapters 5 and 6 or look at the exercises below to help you decide.

    _____

Have you ever watched a tragic movie or read a sad news story and felt worse about your life or the state of the world generally? That is because emotions and thoughts influence each other, just as the CBT diagram in chapter 1 shows. The previous section, "Change Perspective," focused on changing your emotions by changing your thoughts. Sometimes it's easier to work in the other direction, by targeting emotions in order to change thoughts or just feel better in general. For example, if you're thinking that your pain will always feel this bad, it makes sense that despair is the resulting emotion. Similarly, if you're in a state of despair, you're more likely to have thoughts related to hopelessness (*I'll always feel this bad*).

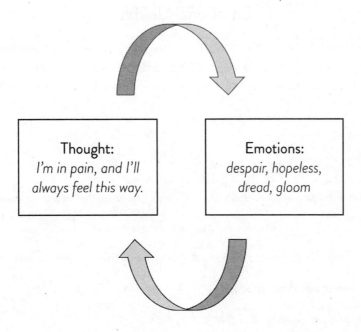

The purpose of the next exercise is to find activities that lead to emotional uplifts. If your emotion shifts even a little from despair or sadness, more hopeful thoughts and emotions tend to follow.

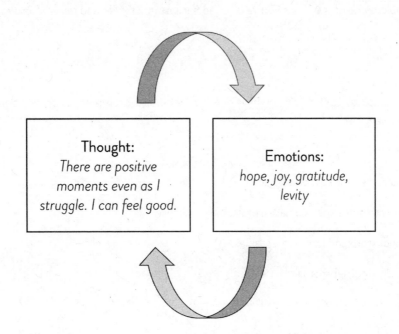

Emotional Uplifts

Read through this list of emotional uplifts below and circle the ones you want to try (aim for five or more). There are also spaces to add your own. Discovering what works best for you is a process—thank you for being flexible as you try these out. If you find something is having a negative effect on your mood or mindset, move on to another option.

- Listen to a song you love.

- Watch or play a sport you enjoy.

- Sit somewhere with interesting scenery (e.g., a body of water, street art, unique buildings).

- Listen to a podcast or an audiobook that lifts your mood.

- Take pictures of things that you would normally just pass by (e.g., flowers, trees).

- List three positive things about yourself.

- Do something on your to-do list and then check it off.

- Call a friend.

- Meet up with someone whom you feel good around.

- Think about some of the times you've laughed hardest in your life and revisit those memories.

- Dance.

- Sing.

- Engage in a spiritual practice if you have one (e.g., meditate, pray, read scripture, contact clergy, attend a religious service).

- Write a poem.

- Volunteer to help people or animals.

- Catch up with someone you haven't talked to in a while.

- Sit in a bookstore and look at magazines.

- Look up silly internet memes.

- Get some exercise, even if it's brief.

- Text a friend about something you have in common.

- Think of a happy memory.

- Watch a funny movie.

- Read a favorite book.

- Go to a live music performance.

- Cook a meal that you enjoy.

- Pet an animal and focus on the softness of their fur.

- Hug someone you love.

- Drink hot coffee or tea.

- Play a musical instrument.

- Think about compliments people have given you.

- Read inspirational quotes or sayings.

- Take a scenic drive.

- Go for a bike ride.

- Watch a favorite television show.

- Plan out a fun activity for the next week.

- Look up new recipes to try.

- Color.

- Do a crossword puzzle.

- Play a tabletop, computer, or video game.

- Daydream about being in your favorite place.

- Make art.

- Read through old cards and letters that people have given to you.

- Read nice messages people wrote in your yearbook.

- Go to a museum in person or look at virtual exhibits.

- Go through the pictures in your phone and spend time looking at your favorites.

- Write a letter or card to someone you care about.

- Write in your journal.

- Put on your favorite outfit.

- Do your hair.

- Paint your nails.

- Eat food from your favorite restaurant.

- Learn something new.

- Read a comic book.

- Go for a swim.

- Do a craft (e.g., knit, scrapbook, sew).

- Make a playlist of uplifting songs.

- Make lists of your favorite things (e.g., movies, shows, bands, actors, restaurants, places).

- Change the way parts of your home look. Add some new lights, a new candle, or a new picture that you find soothing.

- _____

- _____

- _____

- _____

- _____

Is your emotional pain interfering with enjoyment of these activities? You can try increasing your focus on the pleasant parts by using some of the mindfulness exercises in chapter 6. It may also be helpful to view uplifts as tools for improving moments rather than ways to eliminate pain. The experience of uplifts helps us see that we can have moments of joy that exist alongside our pain—sparks of hope for a future that feels better.

Your suicidal thoughts may have started because you felt like you couldn't stand the pain anymore. Most people with suicidal thoughts don't kill themselves, in part, because the intensity of their pain lessens with the passing of time. Even if that intensity later returns in full force, knowing that the suffering will decrease makes it feel more tolerable. You know that you won't have to withstand the worst pain indefinitely. You can see whether this fits with your experiences by tracking your mood with a chart like that in the exercise on the next page.

Track Changes in Emotional Intensity

Select the time period you are tracking and fill that in on the top line (aim for at least fifteen- to thirty-minute increments between recordings). Mark an *X* to indicate the level of pain intensity you're experiencing at each time point. This first chart is filled in as an example.

TIME ↔

PAIN LEVEL ↕	T1 8:00a	T2 8:30a	T3 9:00a	T4 9:30a	T5 10:00a	T6 10:30a	T7 11:00a	T8 11:30a	T9 12:00p	T10 12:30p
10 (worst pain imaginable)	X	X								
9			X	X						
8					X					
7						X				
6							X			
5								X		
4									X	
3										X
2										
1										
0 (no pain)										

Now fill in your own chart.

TIME ↔

PAIN LEVEL ↕	T1	T2	T3	T4	T5	T6	T7	T8	T9	T10
10 (worst pain imaginable)										
9										
8										
7										
6										
5										
4										
3										
2										
1										
0 (no pain)										

After charting your mood, I hope you'll see that there are times when the most unbearable pain lessens. Seeing that there's relief ahead can make it more manageable to persist in those hardest moments. If you can identify what made your mood worse or better, you will also have new ideas about how to prepare for and cope with your ups and downs. For example, if you notice that you feel worse or better after going on social media or hanging around particular people, you can adjust the amount of time spent on those activities. Sometimes the simple passage of time—even without doing anything else—is enough to decrease the intensity. (A copy of the chart is available on the New Harbinger website for downloading and printing, so you can do the exercise multiple times, focusing on different stressors: http://www.newharbinger.com/47025.)

When you're feeling hopeless, it's hard to remember your reasons for living and the coping skills you have for soothing distress. A hope kit (also called a hope box or survival kit; Bryan and Rudd, 2018; Wenzel et al., 2009) is a place to put reminders that you can easily access in times of need. The hope kit can be in a physical box (like a shoe box) or a folder on your phone or computer, and there is also a phone app—Virtual Hope Box (Bush et al., 2014; Denneson et al., 2019).

Make a Hope Kit

In your hope kit, include pictures of people or places, a list of goals, inspirational quotes, your crisis card from chapter 4, songs, poems, copies of exercises you have found helpful in this workbook or in therapy, links to online relaxation exercises, reminders of healthy coping strategies, and anything else that builds hope. Below is an example and then space to design your own hope kit.

Paul's Hope Kit

- a picture of his daughter and wife, his main reasons for living

- a picture of his grandfather, who inspires him

- a picture of friends from his birthday dinner to remind him that he's not alone

- his favorite devotional readings

- a picture of the ocean to remind him of an upcoming trip

- lyrics to songs he finds uplifting:

  - "Keep on Livin'" by Le Tigre

  - "Skeleton Key" by Dessa

  - "Joy" by Against Me!

  - "Feeling Good" by Nina Simone

  - "All the Beauty in This Whole Life" by Brother Ali

- his favorite Black Panther comic book

- a funny meme from The Office

- his crisis plan summary

- a sticker that says, "This too shall pass."

- a list of problem-solving steps

What will go in your hope kit? Make a list below. As you try out different things, you'll find what works best for you. You can adjust the contents of the hope kit accordingly.

- _____

- _____

- _____

- _____

- _____

- _____

- _____

- _____

- _____

- _____

- _____

- _____

By working through this chapter, you have learned the skills from the HOPE acronym: seek Help, find Optimism, change Perspective, and attend to Emotions. When you feel hopeless and the world seems dark, you will always have these tools to create sparks of light. If you still feel hopeless here at the end of this chapter, please don't give up. Give yourself time to retry these exercises, especially the section about seeking help from others. Hold on, be kind to yourself, and allow more space for hope to emerge. Congratulate yourself for finding pieces of hope in small ways and moments. Those little moments can add up over time and light up your life.

Summary of Key Points

- When people want to end their lives, it's often because they do not think their lives will get better.

- You can build hope by seeking help, finding reasons for optimism, changing your perspective, and attending to your emotions.

- Take the knowledge you've found through completing these exercises and build a hope kit that you can lean on when you're feeling hopeless.

Reflection

What thoughts, ideas, and feelings did you have while reading and working through this chapter? Were there certain parts you didn't relate to? What parts did you relate to most? What did you learn?

CHAPTER 8

Strengthen Relationships

As I sat down at my desk to write this chapter, my aunt called. I thought, *How sweet of her to reach out, but I really need to work on this book.* My aunt and I stay connected through social media and only talk on the phone or in person a few times a year, so it was special that she called. Still, I had to write the chapter with the time I carved out during the weekend, so I told her that I'd have to call her back. I sat down, glanced at my outline for strengthening relationships, and prepared to type. Immediately I realized that I was doing the opposite of what I'm about to advise you to do: prioritize your relationships as important components of your health. Make time for them. Let them rise to the same level of importance as getting enough sleep, eating vegetables, and quitting smoking. Research backs me up on how important social connections are to our well-being (Holt-Lunstad et al., 2015), so I decided to make sure my own behavior did too. I called my aunt back right away, and it brightened my mood and energized me. Relationships are always important for our mental health, and this is especially true when you're having suicidal thoughts.

A Look at Your Relationships

Have you found yourself in moments like the one I just described, in which part of you feels like connecting with people, and another part is reluctant for some reason? Are there times when you get a text or the phone rings and you know that you'll feel better if you talk to someone, but you hold back because you feel too tired, busy, or anxious? Take some time to reflect on your general feelings about the relationships in your life.

- Are you lonely right now?

- Do you feel overwhelmed with social commitments?

- Do you feel stuck in toxic relationships?

- Do you feel nourished by the relationships in your life?

Great work reflecting on your current connections with others! Next, start exploring why you feel the way that you do.

- If you're happy with your current social situation, what are you doing that is working?

- If you're unhappy with your social situation, what's getting in the way of making it better?

How are you feeling after reflecting on your relationships? If you're disappointed with your level of social support right now, you might feel sad. Some people don't have as many friends as they would like, while others have friends but don't feel as close to them as they would like. If that is how you feel, try not to blame yourself. Please know that you are worthy of connection and love. This struggle is not a reflection of your value as a person. Many people find it challenging to develop and maintain the relationships they want at different times in their lives.

Though it may be hard to explore your feelings about this, it's important to take the time for it. Loneliness and social isolation are common experiences for people who have suicidal thoughts (Klonsky et al., 2016; Stickley and Koyanagi, 2016; Van Orden et al., 2010). Addressing this is part of the path to making your life better. If you're feeling lonely and isolated right now, I want you to know that we'll work together in this chapter to find ways to feel more supported. I have seen many therapy patients begin our sessions with few friends and few healthy relationships. It's amazing to see them build more connections in their lives through the steps I'm about to walk you through. If they can do it, so can you. I believe in you.

Let's take a deeper look at your current satisfaction with relationships. There will be a worksheet to guide you and an example.

Chloe has always been a shy, introverted person. She grew up in a suburban neighborhood in California, where she had at least three to four close friends who shared her interests in art, music, and books. She also had a close family that did a lot of activities together: cooking, baking, playing cards, and watching movies.

After graduating from college, she moved to Illinois to start a new job. She and her partner tried to make a long-distance relationship work, but it ended when they both decided that it was too hard. Chloe remained in touch with her friends in California mostly through social media interactions and missed them a lot. She would see pictures of them all doing things together and felt sad to be missing out. Chloe also felt embarrassed that they were doing such exciting things, while she was mostly staying at home and watching television on the weekends.

She had friendly coworkers, but they tended to enjoy things that Chloe didn't (like going to crowded bars). Chloe was friendly with a few of her neighbors, but they were busy on the weekends with their children and families. Sometimes they invited her over for dinner, and she would make up an excuse not to go. She felt like they were just being polite and didn't really want her to be there.

Chloe felt lonely and wished she had never moved. She blamed herself for her loneliness and started to think there was something wrong with her. Whenever her family called her, she always said she was doing fine, because she didn't want to burden them with the depression and sadness she was feeling. Chloe felt disappointed in herself. Making friends had been much easier when she was in school. She felt helpless about changing her situation. She wanted to make changes and started with the worksheet below.

My Current Connections (Chloe's Example)

How lonely do you feel on a scale of 0 (not lonely at all) to 10 (extremely lonely)? __7__

If you rated yourself as feeling lonely, what areas do you feel most lonely in?

- ☑ friends who live near me

- ☐ overall friendships

- ☑ romantic relationships

- ☐ family

- ☑ at work

- ☐ other _____

Think about a time when you felt less lonely. What was different then? Is there anything to learn from that time that you could apply to your life now?

When I lived in California, close to my family and friends from college, I had people to go to art museums and out to dinner with. I knew my friends liked being around me and knew the real me. We were all in the same kind of phase in our lives.

What steps can you take to feel less lonely? Include every possibility that comes to mind, even if you decide not to do it later. This is a time for brainstorming.

- I could try going on dating apps to meet people.

- I could try going out with my coworkers even though I don't like bars.

- I could try to meet some new people other than my neighbors.

- Maybe I could move back home to California.

How motivated do you feel to make these changes on a scale of 0 (not at all) to 10 (extremely)? __7__

If you picked anything other than 0, why is that?

I feel sad, and while I like some quiet time on weekends, at other times, I hate it. When I see something cool going on in town, I wish I could have someone to share it with. Sometimes I go a whole weekend without seeing another person. It makes me feel like I'm the only one who can't figure out how to make friends ... like there's something really wrong with me.

How confident do you feel about making those changes on a scale of 0 (not at all) to 10 (extremely)? __3__

If you picked anything other than 0, why is that?

I used to have friends. I have dated people in the past. Maybe it could be like that again. Other people figure out ways to do it, so maybe I can too.

What could get in the way of making changes?

I'm nervous about getting rejected if I try to hang out with more people. If I try and fail, I might feel worse. I'm scared to tell my family and friends back home that I want to talk to them and see them more. They might think I'm too needy or might judge me. Or maybe they have better things to do.

Now that you have read through Chloe's example, please fill out this worksheet for yourself. The first step for working on your loneliness is to examine the sources that exist in your life right now.

My Current Connections

How lonely do you feel on a scale of 0 (not lonely at all) to 10 (extremely lonely)? _____

If you rated yourself as feeling lonely, what areas do you feel most lonely in?

- ☐ friends that live near me

- ☐ overall friendships

- ☐ romantic relationships

- ☐ family

- ☐ at work

- ☐ other _____

Think about a time when you felt less lonely. What was different then? Is there anything to learn from that time that you could apply to your life now?

_____

_____

_____

_____

What steps can you take to feel less lonely? Include every possibility that comes to mind, even if you decide not to do it later.

_____

_____

_____

_____

_____

How motivated do you feel to make these changes on a scale of 0 (not at all) to 10 (extremely)? _____

If you picked anything other than 0, why is that?

_____

_____

_____

How confident do you feel about making those changes on a scale of 0 (not at all) to 10 (extremely)? _____

If you picked anything other than 0, why is that?

_____

_____

_____

What could get in the way of making changes?

_____

_____

_____

How do you feel after filling that out? I hope you feel clearer about the sources of your loneliness and a sense of how you can address them. You might have had the urge to avoid thinking about your loneliness as you filled out the worksheet. If you found that you did have to avoid some of the prompts—or even if you couldn't fill out most of it—don't worry. This is difficult work. Work through the rest of the chapter anyway; it might give you a glimmer of hope and allow you to come back and finish this exercise. And remember that you can look back at that list of confidence boosters in chapter 1 any time you need extra encouragement. And if you stuck with this exercise and finished it even though it was painful—or finished it on a second try—that is a reason to feel proud. You're doing a wonderful job working on these challenging parts of improving your life. Take some time to recognize your strengths and efforts and know that I'm cheering you on!

How Do I Strengthen My Relationships?

Let's start with ways you can strengthen the relationships you already have in your life, since most people find that less intimidating than creating new relationships. There are people Chloe used to feel close to in her life: her family and friends back in California. She is also friendly with some neighbors and coworkers but has not formed more than casual relationships with them. She made a list of them in the example below.

Strengthen Relationships (Chloe's Example)

- Keiko (college friend)

- Mom

- Evelyn (cousin)

- Sebastian (neighbor)

- Brian (coworker)

- Hannah (coworker)

Strengthening Relationships

Look at your life: What relationships do you see that could potentially be strengthened? Try to keep an open mind and include all ideas at this stage. List the people who come to mind who are kind to you. Resist ruling people out at this stage because of a fear of rejection, your assumptions about their interest in being friends, or a seeming lack of common interests.

- _____
- _____
- _____
- _____
- _____
- _____

Did you come up with at least a few people? Great! The next step is to set some small goals to increase contact with the people on the list. Chloe chose to call her mom and tell her that she's been feeling lonely. She plans to tell her mom that she wants to talk at least once a week. Chloe also set a goal of asking her coworker, Hannah, if she wants to try a new restaurant near work for lunch. Chloe's plans are useful steps forward because they are (1) realistic, (2) within her control, and (3) include specific actions.

Now let's look at your list. Can you pick a starting goal to reach out to one or two people in the next few weeks? To begin, you might send a text or an email, make a phone call, or start a conversation. You do not need to set a huge goal to start with because little increases in contact can make a powerful difference in how connected you feel. Write out your goals below.

Person	Action to strengthen relationship	When I will do this

When it comes to strengthening relationships, start with small steps and gradually work your way up to the bigger steps. Below is a worksheet to set your goals over the next month to decrease loneliness. If you get stuck, look at the pages right after it for a list of common obstacles and tips on working through them. Chloe's list appears first as an example.

Relationship Goals (Chloe's example)

Week 1:

- Catch up with Evelyn through a video call and make plans to visit each other.

- Call Keiko (who is extraverted) for advice about making new friends.

Week 2:

- Bring some cookies to Sebastian's family the next time I bake.

- Accept my neighbors' next invitation for dinner.

Week 3:

- Accept my coworkers' invitation to happy hour the next time they ask. If I don't enjoy it, I can suggest another location the next time.

Week 4:

- Start a conversation with Brian about a new art exhibition in town. If he seems interested, invite him to come with me.

Relationship Goals

Week 1:

_____

_____

Week 2:

_____

_____

Week 3:

_____

_____

Week 4:

_____

_____

Possible Obstacles

Did you get stuck while trying to do the previous exercise? Below are some common obstacles that people face as they work to expand their social support and connections. Each obstacle has some suggestions for overcoming it. I hope that you find them helpful as you seek to strengthen relationships.

- *I don't know what I should pick as a goal.* If you're not sure where to start, you can select an action from the list below. You can always update your goals in future weeks if you think of something that fits better with your life then. The purpose is to keep working on strengthening those connections by selecting steps that are practical and helpful to you. The most important goals are to reduce loneliness and social isolation. Use your judgment about healthy people that you feel good interacting with or that you would like to know better. Here are some possible choices:

  - Text a friend or relative and tell them about something that happened in your life.

  - Send an email to a coworker sharing an article you found interesting.

  - Ask an acquaintance you'd like to get to know better if they want to meet for a cup of coffee.

  - Invite someone to watch a movie with you.

  - Send a friend request to an acquaintance on social media, or just follow them.

  - Schedule a call to catch up with someone you haven't talked to in a while.

  - Compliment a coworker about something positive they did at work.

  - Strike up a conversation with your neighbor the next time you see them.

  - Ask a coworker if they want to eat lunch together.

  - When you see a coworker in the break room, ask them how their week has been going.

  - Reconnect with a friend you lost touch with.

  - Call a relative and make plans to visit each other.

  - Invite a relative to play a game with you (either online or in person).

  - Plan to tell your partner that you have been feeling lonely.

  - Plan a date with your partner.

- Ask your partner if you can have ten minutes each night before bed to talk about how your days went.

- Talk to your roommate about the high and low points of their day and then tell them yours.

- Ask a friend who watches the same television show as you if they want to watch it together and talk about it afterward.

- Pick a friend or family member that you trust. Confide in them about your struggles with loneliness. Tell them you'd appreciate it if they could listen to you without judgment or giving advice.

- Pick a relative, friend, or acquaintance who has a social life like the one you want and ask them if they could give you some advice.

- *I'm too nervous.* If you picked your goals but feel too anxious to go through with them, try the following:

  - Start with a smaller goal that you find less intimidating (e.g., start a conversation with a coworker instead of inviting them to do something with you). You can work your way up to the more challenging goals after building some confidence with the ones that you find easier.

  - Use the CBT techniques in chapter 5 to push back on negative thoughts about yourself, worries about what others think of you, or the likelihood that something bad will happen and that you won't be able to cope with it.

  - Plan out what you want to say to the person and then practice saying it until you feel more comfortable. You can practice role-playing the situation with a friend, a therapist, or on your own to make it less anxiety provoking.

  - Revisit chapter 6 and approach yourself with self-compassion and encouragement. It's understandable that you feel nervous. You may have had bad past experiences, or you may be out of practice with socializing. It's okay to feel the way that you do. Even though you're nervous, you can still act bravely to meet your goals. Gently encourage yourself to work on your goals, despite the anxiety. You can do this! You are worthy of the joy that comes from strengthened social connections.

- *The person said no.* Most of us are afraid of rejection. It's natural to want to avoid risking any possible rejection. This becomes especially true if we ask someone to do something, and they decline or otherwise express disinterest. If this happens to you, it's important to know that all people experience rejection at times. It doesn't mean there is something wrong with you. The person could be going through their own difficult circumstances now, you two could just not be a good fit, or maybe the timing isn't right. There are a lot of possible explanations, and none of them amounts to you being unlovable, unlikable, or doing the wrong thing. Give yourself credit for trying—that is what you can control. You cannot control how the person responds. You might feel more anxious about asking the next person to do something, but it's important to try to connect with someone else. You can make that your goal for next week. Revisit the section above if you're feeling nervous and want some help coping with that.

- *Something interfered with the plans (e.g., someone got sick, too busy with work, bad weather).* Here again, the reality is that some parts are not within your control, but I hope you feel proud of yourself for persisting. These kinds of situations happen to everyone from time to time. It's not a sign that you are destined to not have plans work out. Try to plan a new goal for this week or the next. I hope nothing interferes this time, but this chapter is about trying again and again until something works out. This is why I was glad I chose to take the phone call from my aunt that I talked about at the beginning of this chapter. It was worth it to take that opportunity to connect.

I hope that you find this goal-setting framework useful. I offer these suggestions and tools to help you navigate this time in your life, but I want to point out that the most important part is not that you follow exactly what the worksheets say. The vital point of this chapter is that if you work—even in small ways—on strengthening your social connections, your mental health is very likely to improve. These exercises are designed to encourage you to view connections with others as part of your life plan for health and wellness. We need people for support and companionship, and you are deserving of that, even as you struggle.

How Do I Create New Relationships?

Excellent work reading about setting goals and thinking through strategies for enhancing your existing relationships! Now, let's focus on creating new relationships. Chloe said that she'd like to date again and also meet some people who share her artistic interests. Creating brand-new relationships can take more work and even more energy when you're feeling down. I recommend starting with one or two goals per month for meeting new people but select the pace that works for you. For example, Chloe might choose to enroll in a painting class or join a dating app to establish new connections.

What goal would you like to set for yourself for creating new relationships? Remember to be realistic, be specific, and focus on what you can control. If you're not sure what to do, here are some suggestions. Circle at least one or two that you're willing to try.

- Find a meet-up in your community of people who share one of your interests (e.g., writing, hiking, art, billiards, running, knitting, weightlifting, politics, chess).

- Join a dating website or app.

- Join a book club.

- Enroll in a class (e.g., cooking, photography, improv).

- Start a conversation with someone at a coffee shop.

- Attend spiritual services.

- Attend an activity at a house of worship (e.g., Bible study).

- Attend an exercise class and initiate a conversation with someone afterward.

- Join a group that advocates for a cause you believe in.

- Volunteer for a group that is organizing a charity event.

- Join a social media group and start or add to the discussion.

- Check your local comic book or hobby store for game nights that you can join.

- Go to a concert by yourself and talk to the people next to you.

- Join a community choir.

- Join a recreational sports league or martial arts class.

Did you find one or two ideas above that you can aim to act on in the next month? Great!

You have already completed the first step toward forming new connections! Following through with the actions can be tricky for at least two reasons: (1) it can be hard to motivate yourself to get out and meet new people when you're feeling bad about yourself, and (2) when you're feeling down or disconnected, it can be especially hard to put yourself in social situations where you know you'll feel nervous.

In addition to picking realistic goals, it's useful to remember the reasons why you are interested in meeting new people in the first place. For Chloe, she doesn't want to feel so lonely and isolated. She wants her life to be filled with more joy. She wants people to share her thoughts, interests, and feelings with. Think about your reasons for wanting to form new relationships. Make a list of them to put somewhere prominent (e.g., your phone, on a piece of paper on the fridge) so that you can look at it any time you need a motivation boost. For example, Chloe's list looks like this:

My Reasons for Wanting to Meet New People (Chloe's Example)

- I want someone who I can go to the movies or go out to dinner with.

- I want to talk to people who are interested in the same things as me.

- I want to process my daily concerns and thoughts with someone.

- It would be nice to have a partner or at least go out on some dates again.

- I'm sick of feeling lonely and sad every weekend.

- I feel more like myself when I'm sharing my thoughts with others instead of keeping everything in my head.

My Reasons for Wanting to Meet New People

- _____
- _____
- _____
- _____
- _____
- _____
- _____

Cognitive-Behavioral Therapy Helps with Obstacles

The second obstacle I mentioned is that it's hard to socialize when you feel bad about yourself or nervous about being judged. To address this hurdle, let's talk about ideas that come from CBT. The first is that if you're feeling down, depressed, or anxious, your mind and body tell you to avoid, withdraw, and treat yourself poorly (e.g., through negative thoughts, low energy, panic). If you revisit the CBT model in chapter 1, you'll see that you can influence behaviors by changing your thoughts and that you can influence your thoughts by changing your behaviors. According to CBT, one way to feel less down, depressed, or anxious is to _act as if_ you don't feel that way by approaching activities as though you feel confident.

With self-compassion, recognize that those anxious and depressed feelings are painful and make it extra-difficult to meet new people. It's hard to take active approaches to feeling better when you're glum and worried. After acknowledging that it's hard, take some actions (no matter how small) to have fun and meet new people anyway. Chances are that it will lift your mood and increase your confidence over time. Sometimes this happens right away, and other times it takes a while. Hang in there as you make these changes. Both my work as a therapist and my psychology research demonstrate that pleasant activities tend to decrease depression symptoms and improve your mood (Dimidjian et al., 2006). Many feel skeptical about it at first—at least until they try it and start feeling the results. The key is to be persistent and patient with yourself. Encourage yourself to keep taking steps that move you toward your goals while allowing yourself plenty of room for growth and setbacks.

The other CBT idea to keep in mind is that people _habituate_ to—they get used to—situations over time with repeated exposure to them. This means that you might feel highly anxious the first time you attend a new social event, but it's completely natural to feel that way when you're trying something new. Both research (Cuijpers et al., 2016) and my experiences with patients show that the anxiety tends to decrease even during the first exposure to what you fear (e.g., the first time you attend a new social event) and between exposures to what you fear (you'll feel less nervous at the beginning of each subsequent event you attend as you get used to this new activity). It's crucial to give yourself credit for each goal that you meet. The goal is simply to attend social events and stay until your anxiety decreases by at least half (ideally). The goal is not to have a "perfect" experience. Reward yourself for going with self-encouragement or treating yourself to something you enjoy.

I hope you have found this chapter helpful for providing tools and strategies for strengthening the connections in your life. Try to be flexible and open to new ideas as you build and enhance the relationships in your life. Relationships make life more enjoyable and stress more bearable, and they improve your health. I have worked with many people who struggle with isolation and self-hatred but find their way out of it with repeated efforts like those described in this chapter. You can do it too. I believe in you!

Summary of Key Points

- People who have suicidal thoughts often feel lonely or dissatisfied in their relationships with others.

- You can improve your connections by strengthening existing relationships and developing new ones.

- You can pace yourself and set goals to pursue the relationships you want with others.

Reflection

What thoughts, ideas, and feelings did you have while reading and working through this chapter? Were there certain parts you didn't relate to? What relationships do you most want to strengthen—or create—and why?

CHAPTER 9

Make Meaning

In chapter 2, you read that it was common for people to have suicidal thoughts without acting on them. Even in the face of pain and hopelessness, people choose to live when they have meaning in their lives. Because you're reading this book, I'm guessing that you have both reasons for wanting to die and reasons for wanting to live. Even though it may feel confusing, those types of thoughts and emotions often coexist. All of us have emotions and thoughts that are complicated and that don't fit neatly into either-or boxes. The purpose of this chapter is to guide you through making sense of your emotions and thoughts about the meaning in your life.

Reasons for Living

When you're feeling suicidal, the reasons for dying may be louder in your mind. It is useful to identify your reasons for living, so that you can amplify them the next time you're feeling suicidal. As a therapist, I have heard people say that they want to live to see their children grow up. I have also heard people say they want to live to see what the future looks like. People have all kinds of reasons for choosing to stay alive, and there is no judgment in this space about your personal reasons for wanting to live.

Reasons for Living Inventory

[Adapted from the appendix in *Building a Life Worth Living: A Memoir* by Marsha M. Linehan, copyright © 2020 by Dr. Marsha M. Linehan. Used by permission of Random House, an imprint and division of Penguin Random House LLC. All rights reserved.]

The Reasons for Living Inventory is printed below. Please circle any of the forty-seven statements that are true for you right now, and then add any reasons you have for living that you do not see on the list. If you circle a statement with a question next to it, please respond to the question.

Survival and Coping Beliefs

1. I care enough about myself to live.

2. I believe I can find other solutions to solve my problems.

3.   I still have many things left to do. *Please list what they are here:*

_____

_____

_____

_____

4.   I have hope that things will improve and the future will be happier.

5.   I have the courage to face life.

6.   I want to experience all that life has to offer, and there are many experiences I haven't had yet that I want to have. *Write what they are here:*

_____

_____

_____

_____

7.   I believe everything has a way of working out for the best.

8.   I believe I can find a purpose in life, a reason to live.

9.   I have a love of life.

10.   No matter how badly I feel, I know that it will not last.

11.   Life is too beautiful and precious to end it.

12.   I am happy and content with my life.

13.   I am curious about what will happen in the future.

14.   I see no reason to hurry death along.

15.   I believe I can learn to adjust or cope with my problems.

16.   I believe that killing myself would not really accomplish or solve anything.

17.   I have a desire to live.

18.   I am too stable to kill myself.

19. I have future plans that I am looking forward to carrying out. *What are they?*

_____

_____

_____

_____

20. I do not believe that things get miserable or hopeless enough that I would rather be dead.

21. I do not want to die.

22. Life is all we have and is better than nothing.

23. I believe I have control over my life and destiny.

Responsibility to Family

24. It would hurt my family too much. *Who would feel most hurt? How would they feel if you died by suicide ?*

_____

_____

_____

_____

25. I would not want my family to feel guilty afterward.

26. I would not want my family to think I was selfish or a coward. *Please note that suicidal thoughts do not mean you are selfish or a coward, but I have included all of the items on this inventory because people experiencing suicidal thoughts have listed them as reasons for living.*

27. My family depends on me and needs me. *Who depends on you?*

_____

_____

_____

_____

28. I love and enjoy my family too much and could not leave them.

29. My family might believe I did not love them.

30. I have a responsibility and commitment to my family.

Child-Related Concerns

31. The effect of on my children would be harmful. *How would dying by suicide harm your children?*

_____

_____

_____

_____

32. It would not be fair to leave the children to others to take care of.

33. I want to watch the children as they grow. *What do you look most forward to seeing? What would you miss out on?*

_____

_____

_____

_____

Fear of Suicide

34. I am afraid of the actual *act* of killing myself (the pain, blood, violence).

35. I am a coward and do not have the guts to do it.

36. I am so inept that my method would not work.

37. I am afraid that my method of killing myself would fail.

38. I am afraid of the unknown.

39. I am afraid of death.

40. I could not decide where, when, and how to do it.

Fear of Social Disapproval

41. Other people would think I am weak and selfish.

42. I would not want people to think that I did not have control over my life.

43. I am concerned about what others would think of me.

Moral Objections

> 44. My religious beliefs forbid it.
>
> 45. I believe only God has the right to end life.
>
> 46. I consider it morally wrong.
>
> 47. I am afraid of going to hell.

Other Reasons for Living

- _____
- _____
- _____
- _____

After looking through the list, what are your top three reasons for living right now? List them below:

My Most Important Reasons for Living

1. _____
2. _____
3. _____

Do other important reasons for living come to mind? Add them below.

- _____
- _____
- _____
- _____

Find Meaning

How did you feel during that exercise? Did you struggle to find reasons for living or did they come easily to you? If you struggled, it may be because your life feels empty right now. I want you to know that it's not because you're doing something wrong. It just means that you need a little help finding what fulfills you.

All of us need help with that at times. In fact, people have been trying to understand the purpose of existence for thousands of years, often looking to religion, science, art, and philosophy to find answers. Where have you found answers in the past? Those same sources may help you regain your sense of meaning right now.

> "For the meaning of life differs from man to man, from day to day and from hour to hour. What matters, therefore, is not the meaning of life in general but rather the specific meaning of a person's life at a given moment." —Victor Frankl, *Man's Search for Meaning*

The beauty of Frankl's quote is that he says that you can learn the skills for pursuing meaning at a given moment in your life and revisit the process any time that you need it. This chapter focuses on teaching you the steps of that meaning-making process. First, I'll describe some of Frankl's background and the reason why he wrote *Man's Search for Meaning* (1955). Frankl experienced excruciating emotional and physical pain while imprisoned by the Nazis in concentration camps. His family, including his parents, brother, and wife, who died during the Holocaust. In the concentration camps, Frankl was surrounded by people who talked about suicide. He made a commitment to himself that he wouldn't end his life, despite the suffering and hopelessness he faced. Frankl described how his connection to a specific project became a reason for wanting to survive.

Arriving at Auschwitz, his clothes and possessions were taken from him, including a manuscript he was writing. The desire to rewrite that manuscript one day drew him to life. After liberation, he completed that project, and he said that the meaning of his life became helping others find the meaning in theirs. When people identify meaning in their lives as Frankl did, their suicide risk tends to be lower (Bryan et al., 2019).

Now let's use Frankl's framework to find the specific meaning in your life at this moment. He said that people find purpose (1) by creating a work or doing a deed (actions), (2) through experiences, or (3) through an attitude taken toward unavoidable suffering. If you're feeling overwhelmed, it's important to note that both Frankl and the 3ST state that you only need one of these three types of meaning to prevent suicide. After reading through this chapter, you can decide which type fits best with your life right now, and you can adjust it in the future as your life changes.

Values

Actions tend to be most meaningful when they align with our values. It's not always easy to identify our priorities, because they change over the course of our lives. Let's focus on the values that are most important in your life at this moment. As you look at the list below, think about the following questions:

- What qualities do I admire in others?

- What kind of person do I want to be?

- How do I want others to perceive me?

Mark the values you care most about and then add any that are missing from the list when you are done.

☐ achievement	☐ fun	☐ productivity
☐ advocacy	☐ generosity	☐ rationality
☐ authenticity	☐ gratitude	☐ religion
☐ beauty	☐ hard work	☐ resourcefulness
☐ charity	☐ honor	☐ respect
☐ compassion	☐ humility	☐ responsibility
☐ competence	☐ humor	☐ rigor
☐ courage	☐ inclusiveness	☐ safety
☐ creativity	☐ independence	☐ sensitivity
☐ critical thinking	☐ intellect	☐ service
☐ curiosity	☐ joy	☐ sincerity
☐ dependability	☐ justice	☐ spirituality
☐ dignity	☐ kindness	☐ spontaneity
☐ discipline	☐ knowledge	☐ stability
☐ diversity	☐ love	☐ strength
☐ education	☐ loyalty	☐ success
☐ empathy	☐ openness	☐ toughness
☐ enthusiasm	☐ optimism	☐ tradition
☐ ethics	☐ order	☐ trust
☐ equality	☐ originality	☐ wisdom
☐ fairness	☐ passion	☐ _____
☐ family	☐ patience	☐ _____
☐ fitness	☐ peace	☐ _____
☐ flexibility	☐ perseverance	☐ _____
☐ friendship	☐ popularity	

Great job thinking through your values. If you had to select your top three values, what would they be? Let's go through each in the exercise below and see how they fit into your life currently. When you live a life consistent with your values, you're more likely to find it worth living even in the face of pain. This exercise will help you identify ways to take more actions that are consistent with your values to increase meaning. We'll begin this exercise with an example.

Find Meaning in Actions (Example)

List one of your values below.

knowledge

- What actions do you take in your life that are consistent with this value?

  I try to read articles on topics I'm interested in.

  I watch documentaries.

- What additional actions could you take that are aligned with this value?

  Go to a public talk.

  Visit a museum.

  Attend a cooking class.

- What's a first, realistic step you can take toward acting on that value? No step is too small. The goal is just to move in the direction of acting on your values a bit more to enhance the meaning in your life.

  Find out what exhibits are at the museum in my town.

Now that you've read through the example, let's focus on your values.

Find Meaning in Actions

List your number 1 value below:

_____

- What actions do you take in your life that are consistent with this value?

  _____

  _____

- What additional actions could you take that are aligned with this value?

  _____

  _____

- What's a first, realistic step you can take toward acting on that value? No step is too small. The goal is just to move in the direction of acting on your values a bit more to enhance meaning in your life.

  _____

  _____

List your number 2 value below:

_____

- What actions do you take in your life that are consistent with this value?

  _____

  _____

- What additional actions could you take that are aligned with this value?

  _____

  _____

- What's a first, realistic step you can take toward acting on that value? No step is too small. The goal is just to move in the direction of acting on your values a bit more to enhance meaning in your life.

  _____

  _____

List your number 3 value below:

_____

- What actions do you take in your life that are consistent with this value?

  _____

  _____

- What additional actions could you take that are aligned with this value?

  _____

  _____

- What's a first, realistic step you can take toward acting on that value? No step is too small. The goal is just to move in the direction of acting on your values a bit more to enhance meaning in your life.

  _____

  _____

Meaning Through Experiences

Frankl described this type of meaning as experiencing "goodness, truth, and beauty" through nature, culture, or the love of another person. When you think back on the transformative experiences of your life, what comes to mind? Have any of the following happened to you?

- traveling and seeing new places that give you a stronger sense of the commonalities among all people

- attending a cultural or community event and learning something that led to a profound change in your life

- forming a special connection with a pet or other animal

- if you're spiritual, praying or worship leading to a closeness with a higher power

- caring for someone who is ill and perceiving humanity in a new way

- seeing a movie, book, play, or concert and feeling lifted up by its message

- being out in nature (e.g., a mountain, beach, or forest) and feeling connected with something bigger than yourself

If you're struggling now, it may be hard to find ways to recreate those types of meaningful experiences. I'd like you to spend time thinking about realistic steps you can take to seek out meaning through experiences with nature and cultural events. For example, you might consider volunteering for a charity you care about, attending a spiritual service (if you're a spiritual person), traveling, or connecting with a group that shares one of your passions or interests (e.g., a book club, a political group, a charity event). Making plans for these types of experiences can give you things to look forward to and a sense of purpose. If you are not feeling up to those types of activities, aim for something at a smaller scale: read an engrossing book, watch a documentary on someone whose life inspires you, take a short walk outside, work on a craft or hobby you enjoy, or listen to a moving song.

Find Meaning in Experiences

List five meaningful experiences you will pursue and when you plan to do them.

Experience:	When I Will Try It:

Meaning in Relationships

Now that we have considered nature and cultural experiences, let's think about the relationships that give you the most meaning in your life. Among the most common reasons my patients have for wanting to stay alive is that they do not want to hurt their parents or children. What relationships do you derive the most meaning from right now? If you find that you can't point to current meaning in any of your relationships, write about what you could do to create more meaningful connections in the space below. You may find it helpful to revisit chapter 8 for this exercise. If you have identified relationships that are meaningful but want to make them even more so, list actions you can take to do that. For example, you could:

- dedicate time for more reflection about what you value about that person and share that with them

- list the things about the relationship that you're grateful for

- attend couples therapy to enhance communication

- have a heart-to-heart talk about your feelings about one another

- make plans to talk more or do more fun activities together

Find Meaning in Relationships

Relationship Action:	When I Will Do It:

Meaning in Suffering

Frankl said that the most meaningful act you can do with regard to suffering is to remove or reduce the source of suffering. For those reasons, chapters 5 and 6 focus on strategies to reduce pain through problem solving, CBT, self-compassion, and acceptance. However, some suffering in life is unavoidable. If you are reading this book, you likely know this from firsthand experience. For pain that cannot be alleviated, the goal becomes trying to find meaning in that experience.

Find Meaning in Suffering

Let's start this process by considering an area where you have experienced suffering. What was that experience?

_____

_____

_____

_____

What made the suffering in that experience unavoidable?

_____

_____

_____

_____

Did you find any meaning in that experience or was meaning hard to find?

_____

_____

_____

_____

I'm so sorry that you suffered through those hardships and that you are experiencing this pain now. As you reflect on the kinds of suffering you experienced, there are certain times when it may be easier to find meaning:

- When the suffering was followed by a positive outcome (e.g., sacrifices made at work led to a better position, chemotherapy treatment led to cancer remission, putting someone else first strengthened a relationship).

- When there is some logic to the suffering (e.g., you made a mistake and faced the consequences for it, you know that others in your position had to go through similar obstacles).

It's harder to find meaning in suffering when there seems to be no logic and no obvious positive outcome or when there is missing information as to why the suffering happened (e.g., the sudden death of a loved one, assault, abuse, a romantic partner who is unfaithful, infertility issues, a tragic accident). I want to validate that it takes more effort in those types of situations to find meaning. If you haven't found meaning in those kinds of suffering yet, you're not doing anything wrong. It just takes time—sometimes a long period of time—to feel any other way than hurt. Try to be patient with yourself through the process. In my therapy practice, my patients have found meaning in suffering in different ways. Some of those potential paths to meaning are listed below as examples.

- a change in life priorities and perspectives (e.g., being more "in the moment," caring more for one's own health)

- increased appreciation for other areas of life

- feeling more compassionate and less judgmental of others

- starting, joining, or contributing to an organization that works to prevent the same kind of suffering for others

- sharing the experience publicly, in small groups, or with loved ones to create greater understanding

- creating art, literature, or music inspired by the suffering

- volunteering time to support others who are going through difficult times

- developing new skills to adapt to a difficult situation

- new insight

- strengthened spirituality

- an increased sense of humility

- more generosity and kindness to loved ones

- advocating for one's self and others

- more closeness and intimacy in relationships

- increased assertiveness and boundary setting

- feeling less preoccupied by other people's opinions

- forming new relationships with people who suffered in a similar way

As you read through those examples, did any feel familiar to you? If not, are there any types of meaning that you can try to apply to your own suffering? Start slowly by selecting one that seems most relevant for you. Think about how you can incorporate that into your life and write about it below. If none fit, try to think of your own. As I said above, it takes time to find the pathway that works best for you. Trial and error are often involved. Try to be loving and patient toward yourself as you figure this out.

One way I can try to find meaning in my suffering:

_____

_____

Make a Meaning Collage

In order to tie the different pieces of this chapter together, I recommend creating a meaning collage that will serve as a physical reminder of all the meaningful components of your life. I hope that you have fun with this—it's an opportunity to get creative. Select photos, quotes, pictures, or anything else that represents your goals, reasons for living, values, and meaning in your life. Then, cut them out and glue or tape them onto a poster board or piece of paper. Or you could make a digital meaning collage on your computer. The goal is to enjoy the process and focus on your sense of purpose. It does not have to be a fancy or complicated collage at all. When you're done with this project, you can hang it on your wall, put it in your wallet, take a picture of it with your phone, or put it somewhere else that is easy to access any time you are feeling empty or struggling to find meaning. If it is a digital collage, you could make it the desktop on your computer. This is a tangible way to magnify your reasons for living when the reasons for dying are taking up more space in your mind.

Remember that you can revisit the exercises in this chapter whenever you're struggling to find meaning. You now have the skills to identify your values and take actions that make more meaning in your life. Making meaning in life is hard work, and you're doing an excellent job thinking through these ideas! I hope that you feel empowered through the new knowledge and skills you learned in this chapter.

Summary of Key Points

- When you're in pain and feeling hopeless, a sense of purpose can help you feel more connected to life.

- You can make meaning through actions, in relationships or experiences, and through the attitudes you take toward suffering.

- There are many pathways to creating more meaning in your life. Try to pick a small step as a starting place. Be kind to yourself as you build more meaning in your life.

Reflection

What thoughts, ideas, and feelings did you have while reading and working through this chapter? Were there certain parts you didn't relate to? What parts did you relate to most? What did you learn?

CHAPTER 10

Create Safety

Find a quiet space, if you can, and think about a time when your suicidal feelings were at their most intense. What was going on in your life at the time? It's not uncommon for people who are feeling suicidal to start daydreaming about killing themselves during those times, sometimes in great detail. You might imagine past suicide attempts, how people would respond to your death, or future plans for killing yourself. For some, these experiences are jarring and scary. Others experience a sense of relief and escape. Is this where your mind goes when your suicidal thoughts are most intense?

Research suggests that fantasizing about suicide can lead to temporary relief and mood boosts, but that it makes suicidal desire more intense over time (Selby et al., 2007). That is why I want to make sure to validate your desire to feel better and let you know that you're not alone in having those thoughts, while also working together to identify other options for coping with pain. Your feelings and your life both matter, which is why this chapter prioritizes creating physical and emotional safety during times when you're thinking about suicide. This chapter is organized around examining first physical safety and then emotional safety. It takes you through exercises for coping that don't involve fantasizing about suicide or putting yourself in harm's way in the process.

Reflect on the Past

As you were thinking about times when your suicidal desire was most intense, did memories about a specific suicide attempt come up? Were there other times when you had a strong desire for suicide but did not act on it? Take a moment to think about the differences between those incidents. In therapy, my patients have shared two major factors that make a difference between attempting suicide and not making that attempt when they have severe suicidal desire. They are related to (1) fear (e.g., "I thought about killing myself, but I was too afraid of the pain" or "I didn't know what would happen after I died"), and (2) access to things to hurt themselves with at the time (e.g., "My partner put the gun in a safe, and I didn't have the combination" or "I didn't have enough medication to overdose on and couldn't bring myself to go to the store").

A Protective Survival Instinct

In chapter 3, I explained how the 3ST states that if you are in pain and hopeless and if your pain is greater than your connection to life, you are likely to attempt suicide if you are capable of it. The reasoning behind this is that many people who desire suicide may not be capable of it because of a built-in human instinct to avoid pain and fear death (Van Orden et al., 2010). That survival instinct is lifesaving and can prevent people from ending their lives. Your life is worth saving. If you are struggling to believe that, it is worth revisiting the exercises in chapter 6 that foster self-compassion.

Research shows that creating a safe environment with reduced access to objects that you can use to kill yourself (e.g., locking up medications, storing bullets separate from a gun, putting a barrier on a bridge that prevents falling, removing items that could be used to self-injure) effectively prevents many suicides (Yip et al., 2012). Some believe this is due to the most intense moments of suicidal desire passing or decreasing in the time it would take to access other methods for suicide. Understandably, some people think, *If I don't have access to a gun when I'm in crisis, I'll just find another way to kill myself.* However, the science suggests that many people have a preferred method for suicide and do not seek out another method if the first one is not available. The lack of access can get you through the moment of crisis without self-harm. Secondly, if you don't have access to a gun while suicidal and decide to use another method, the lack of access can still be lifesaving if the second method is less lethal. For these reasons, the focus of this chapter is to collaboratively create safety in those times of crisis.

Know Your Risk Factors

When you're feeling vulnerable, sad, scared, or any other mix of emotions as you consider suicide, it can be hard to keep yourself safe. In those moments, you will be safer if you understand your own capability for suicide and how to reduce it when it really counts. There are three kinds of capability for suicide in the 3ST, which builds on the capability described in the interpersonal theory of suicide: dispositional (mostly genetic—what you're born with, such as a high pain tolerance), acquired (life experiences that make you less afraid of pain and death, such as physical trauma), and practical (knowledge and access to ways of killing yourself, such as knowing how to use a gun). Let's explore how these different types of capability apply to your life, starting with an example.

When Malcolm started college, he found a passion for social justice causes, especially those focused on helping children in poverty. As a basketball player and student, his life was busy, but he prioritized community activism. He loved bonding with others who were working to make the world a better place. With friends, Malcolm cofounded a community garden in a part of his city where many families lived in poverty. He taught children how to grow their own fruit, vegetables, and flowers. Over time, he found that this space allowed the children to open up about their struggles and provided opportunities to give them emotional support.

After Malcolm graduated and began full-time work as a teacher, he struggled to balance the demands of his job and his community activism. He reduced his time in the garden and felt guilty about not being able to contribute. Then he started struggling with severe fatigue. At first, his doctor dismissed his concerns about a medical cause and said that he should work less; another doctor said that it was depression. When he made some life changes and still didn't feel better, he started to lose hope about feeling like himself again. He was ultimately diagnosed with a disease that was treatable but that he would have to live with for the rest of his life.

Malcolm knew that if he wanted to keep teaching, he would have to cut out his work at the garden and other parts of his life. He experienced shame and dread about his future. Malcolm worried he wouldn't be able to be an active, engaged father. He was angry at the early physicians who first overlooked his medical problem. Malcolm was also ashamed to share his medical problem with others, because he worried that they'd treat him differently. Faced with making up for the time lost in the past year and an imagined future where he thought he'd have to sacrifice his dreams and passions, Malcolm started drinking alcohol regularly. He hoped it would dampen the pain, but it intensified his sadness and shame instead.

One night, he thought, "I could just be done with all of this if I take all my pain pills." Malcolm held the bottle of pills in his hand for a few minutes and ended up drifting off to sleep without harming himself. He woke up the next morning and started thinking about ways to create a safer environment so that he would not come so close to harming himself in the future. He had lost a cousin to suicide and remembered how much it had hurt all those left behind. Despite everything, Malcolm had hope that he could find a way to still fulfill his dreams. In order to create a physically safe environment, Malcolm considered different factors and filled out the worksheet below.

Now that you have read through Malcolm's story, let's reflect on the role of capability for suicide in your life so that we better understand your risk factors and safety needs. It can be painful to think about these aspects of your life. Take your time, take breaks as needed, and feel free to reach out for help from someone else if you get stuck.

Capability for Suicide (including Malcolm's Example)

Dispositional

Do you have a high pain tolerance?

Yes. Even as a kid, my parents noticed that I rarely cried or got upset when I got hurt. The pain of self-harm doesn't scare me.

How strong is your fear of death?

I'm scared of dying, because I'm not sure what will happen after I die. I used to think I'd go to heaven, but now I'm not so sure.

Are you related to anyone who has died by suicide or attempted suicide?

My cousin killed himself. My grandfather died in a car accident after being depressed most of his life. My dad wondered if it was truly an accident or intentional.

Do you tend to be impulsive (e.g., seek out risky situations, make rash decisions)?

Not really. I have done things like skydiving and driving my car really fast, but mostly, I sit back and think things through. When I drink too much, I can be impulsive (get in a fight, make bad decisions). I have to watch out for that.

After reflecting on your dispositional capability for suicide, what are some steps you can take to create safety in your life?

After realizing that I have a pretty high threshold for pain, I'm thinking I need to focus on my fear of what will happen after I die when I'm having suicidal thoughts—just to pull my mind back to life. I also need to limit my alcohol use to none or very little for now, so I don't do impulsive things I later regret.

Dispositional

Do you have a high pain tolerance?

_____

_____

How strong is your fear of death?

_____

_____

_____

Are you related to anyone who has died by suicide or attempted suicide?

_____

_____

_____

Do you tend to be impulsive (e.g., seek out risky situations, make rash decisions)?

_____

_____

_____

After reflecting on your dispositional capability for suicide, what are some steps you can take to create safety in your life?

_____

_____

_____

_____

Acquired

Have you had life experiences that made you less afraid of death?

My family life was pretty supportive and stable. Sometimes when I feel down, I notice myself daydreaming about killing myself, especially when I'm drinking. It makes my pain seem worse, like a magnifying glass is being held up to it. When my pain is that bad, I don't feel afraid of death like I do when I'm sober.

What about experiences that made you more tolerant of pain?

As a college basketball player, I had some serious injuries and endured a lot of pain while training and playing.

After reflecting on your acquired capability for suicide, what are some steps you can take to create safety in your life?

I think just recognizing that I have been through some things in my life that make suicide less scary. I can't undo my past, but it's good for me to keep in mind that I have a higher risk than some other people. I also should be careful about my drinking. I usually think it will make me feel better, but it really doesn't. If I do drink, I should limit it to one to two drinks. I can think about some other ways to improve my mood besides daydreaming and planning for suicide. The thing I really want is relief. I can try using some healthier coping skills (e.g., exercise, self-soothing, reaching out to a friend).

Acquired

Have you had life experiences that made you less afraid of death?

_____

_____

_____

What about experiences that made you more tolerant of pain?

_____

_____

After reflecting on your acquired capability for suicide, what are some steps you can take to create safety in your life?

_____

_____

_____

_____

_____

_____

Practical

Do you have knowledge about ways to die by suicide as a result of your profession, hobbies, looking up information, or some other way?

I don't have a gun in my house. When I've been at my lowest points, I have thought about looking into other methods of suicide.

Do you currently have easy access to lethal means? Are there ways that you can make them harder to access when you're at risk for hurting yourself? What are those?

I have medicines for my medical condition. If I start feeling suicidal, I should store them in my basement or give them to a friend to hold on to. If I ever get a gun, I should make sure I take a course on gun safety and consider things like storing the bullets separately.

After reflecting on your practical capability for suicide, what are some steps you can take to create safety in your life?

The big thing for me is to stop myself from looking up information about ways to kill myself. It sometimes gives me a little relief, but it also makes me uneasy when I think about wanting to stay safe. It's better if I don't gain any more knowledge about it and focus on learning other things that lift me up instead (e.g., gardening, history, sports, activism).

Practical

Do you have knowledge about ways to die by suicide as a result of your profession, hobbies, looking up information, or some other way?

_____

_____

Do you currently have easy access to lethal means? Are there ways that you can make them harder to access when you're at risk for hurting yourself? What are those?

_____

_____

_____

After reflecting on your practical capability for suicide, what are some steps you can take to create safety in your life?

_____

_____

_____

_____

_____

You're doing a great job reading and working through these exercises and reflecting on ways to decrease your capability for suicide. These are hard steps, but the work you are doing now is literally lifesaving for many people. I hope you feel proud of yourself for that.

Get Help with Safety Planning

In chapter 8, we talked about how feeling suicidal can make it hard to care for yourself at the times when you're in the most danger of hurting yourself. That is because the feelings and emotional pain can be so overwhelming that they are hard to face on your own. If you're not sure how to increase your physical safety, you can try talking to a therapist or a friend or loved one about it. Make sure to pick someone you trust. In case the words are hard to find, I have provided some sample scripts below.

- "Sometimes I struggle with suicidal thoughts. I want to make sure that I'm safe when that happens. Would you be willing to hold on to my medications until I'm feeling less suicidal? I can let you know when my risk is lower."

- "I'm having thoughts about suicide again, and I have been thinking about using a gun. It's really hard for me to share this with you. I was wondering if you could go with me to get a safe to store my gun in until I'm not feeling suicidal."

- "I'm drinking and using drugs more lately when I feel sad. I think it makes me feel worse. I'm wondering if you could check in with me over the next couple of nights just to see how I'm doing. I think that would help keep me from drinking and using drugs to drown out my thoughts."

I hope that you find these sample scripts helpful for finding the words. If you want to write your own script out, consider the framework below.

- First, think of a person you trust to ask for help with safety.

- Next, identify the specific action you want from them (e.g., storing the methods you're thinking about using, checking in on you, staying with you, or letting you stay at their place).

- Then, come up with a back-up plan if that does not work (e.g., another person, a hotline, a mental health professional, or contacting a mobile crisis unit). Revisit your crisis plan summary as needed.

- After completing these steps, you can fill out this script, if it's helpful.

  "Hi _____ (name). I'm having some thoughts about suicide. I don't want to hurt myself, so I'm thinking of ways to stay as safe as possible. Will you please help me by _____ (name specific action) _____? Thank you."

Substitutes for Daydreaming About Suicide

Before concluding the section on physical safety, let's return to a topic from the beginning of the chapter. If you daydream about suicide, I'd like you to consider the possibility of substitute behaviors like Malcolm did. Below is a list with some alternative, safer ways to use your imagination to find relief and escape. You can make a list of healthy go-to daydreams or nostalgic states you can turn to instead of imagining killing yourself. That way, when the urge arises, you'll have options to cope with your distress.

- imagine your life improving

- reflect on happy memories from the past

- daydream about something you're looking forward to

- daydream by getting absorbed in a book or a movie

- try a relaxation exercise that includes visualizing being somewhere you love (e.g., the beach, a forest, a lake, a particular room, or other location)

- imagine being with someone you love, someone you feel safe around

- _____

- _____

- _____

- _____

Emotional Safety: Learn What Works When You Feel Vulnerable

In the second half of this chapter, we'll identify what you find most helpful when you're feeling suicidal and emotionally vulnerable. It's important to have trusted people who you can share your innermost feelings with in times of need. As we discussed earlier in the book, some people with suicidal thoughts have negative experiences when they ask for help. Sometimes the people around you—even people who care deeply about you—are uncomfortable talking about suicidal thoughts, so they avoid or change the topic if you bring it up. Other times, they might offer advice when you really want them to listen to you. Some people sound judgmental when you open up to them about your feelings (e.g., "it's not that big of a deal" or "your life isn't that rough" or "I just stop thinking like that when I'm down. You can do that too"). This can cause greater pain for you when you're vulnerable. After we reflect on what you need for emotional safety, then we can talk about how you can increase emotional safety in your life.

Think about someone you are comfortable talking to about your feelings. How do you feel in their presence? What is it that they do or don't do that makes you feel safe being vulnerable with them? Now think about someone who you have not felt emotionally safe with. How do you feel in their presence? What is it they do or don't do that makes you feel emotionally unsafe around them? Do they criticize you or ridicule you? Do they interrupt you? Do they turn the conversation to themselves?

Make a Safety Word Cloud

Let's think more about safety by creating a word cloud. You can draw this by hand or use a word cloud maker website. List words or phrases that represent aspects of your physical and emotional safety. The words that mean most to you can appear bigger than the other words in the cloud. The example below is by someone who finds the following most important for safety: "patient with me," "listened to," "not alone." They also listed actions that increase a sense of safety, such as "specific plans," "hug," and "treated as knowledgeable." The cloud includes specific people and settings that feel safe (e.g., Sandy, Matt, Grandma, family dinners, the ocean). After you complete this project, you can save it on your phone or put it in your hope kit as a reminder of when you feel safest.

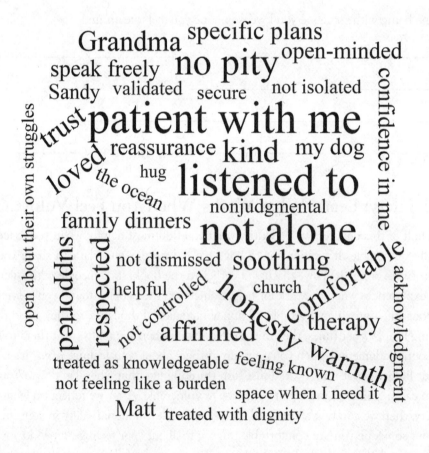

Now that you've thought about what helps when you're feeling emotionally vulnerable, let's explore some of the factors that influence whether you open up to others or not.

Dorothea is a widowed woman in her seventies who did not have any serious mental health struggles until after she retired. Then she started feeling like life was empty and pointless. She found herself thinking about death and not minding the idea that a disease or an accident could end her life at any moment. She tried to fill the void through various activities, but it wasn't enough to make life enjoyable.

Her adult children contact her every week to check in on her. She doesn't want them to worry, so she says she feels fine and that she enjoys the alone time. Dorothea also has a group of friends who meet up weekly for potlucks and card playing. Some of the other women in the group have opened up about their anxiety, depression, and loneliness. Dorothea always listens, but says she feels fine when people ask how she's doing. She likes being a "rock" for people who are going through tough times and feels most comfortable in situations in which she supports others.

Lately, she's started to feel dread about the days ahead instead of her usual optimism. She lies awake at night trying to sleep and searching for a former clarity. Dorothea is anxious about opening up about her feelings but is starting to think she should talk to somebody. She decided to make a list of pros and cons of opening up to people.

Pros and Cons of Opening Up to Others (Dorothea's Example)

Pros:

- I might feel better sharing how I feel.

- I would feel less alone.

- They might have good advice.

- They might invite me to spend more time together.

- They could help me get out of my head and look at things in different ways.

- It could deepen our relationships and make them more like two-way friendships. We could lean on each other.

Cons:

- They could reject me (though this probably won't happen).

- I'll be out of my comfort zone.

- I'll have to face how I really feel instead of trying to avoid it and distract myself.

Do you relate to Dorothea? If you have different pros and cons, it might be helpful to write those out for yourself.

Pros and Cons of Opening Up to Others

Pros:

_____

_____

_____

_____

_____

Cons:

_____

_____

_____

_____

_____

Sharing your feelings can make you more vulnerable to others, but it's hard to cope with stressors on our own. We tend to do better by taking the risk of opening up to the right people. For example, after Dorothea decided to share her feelings, she thought about her approach in more detail. She decided to share her feelings with one person and hoped that would help her be more open with others.

Dorothea chose her son, because he had mentioned that he worried about her. While she didn't want him to worry, she suspected he could already tell her mood had been flat or down when they chatted. She also knew that he was nonjudgmental about mental health issues and had been to therapy for depression.

If you're thinking about opening up about your struggles, who is at the top of your list to talk to? What would you like to say to them and what are you hoping to get from them? Thinking about these things ahead of time makes the process of sharing your feelings go smoother.

You may have different needs from the different people in your life. For example, Dorothea could turn to her son for advice because he had his own mental health problems and thus could relate to her. She could turn to one of the friends she played cards with for validation and understanding about life changes after retirement. This topic can be hard to think about, but you're sticking with it to find more emotional safety in your life. Once you have reflected on what you find helpful and unhelpful from others, it can still be hard and can provoke a lot of anxiety to approach someone about your suicidal thoughts. Some people find that it goes smoother by initially reaching out to the person by text or email. Here are examples to help you figure out how to start a conversation with the person or people you choose.

- "This is hard for me to talk about right now, but I have been feeling stressed lately. I don't want to scare you, but I think I need some help. I'm having thoughts about death. It would help me if I could talk about them with you. I would like you to please listen before jumping in. I don't think advice would be helpful right now, but it would help to be heard. Can you do that for me right now? Thank you."

- "I'm a little nervous to share this, but I have been a bit lonely lately. I'm wondering if I can talk to you about what's on my mind. It would help me just to process my feelings and get input from someone else. My mind feels jumbled right now."

- "I'm wondering if we could meet up for lunch. I have a few things on my mind, and I seem to be stuck. It would help if you just spent time with me. You know me well and might have ideas about how to solve my problems."

- "I'm wondering if we can set up a time to talk about my struggles right now. I have tried praying and solving them on my own, and I'm not feeling any better."

I hope these scripts are helpful for ideas about how to (1) choose someone you trust with your feelings, (2) express what you want to talk to them about (e.g., suicidal thoughts, loneliness, stressors), (3) ask specifically for what you want from them (e.g., to listen, to problem solve, to encourage you), and (4) thank them for helping you and let them know things you've already tried that you did not find helpful.

Summary of Key Points

- Even when people experience suicidal thoughts, there is a survival instinct drawing us toward life and away from the pain and fear of death.

- There are three different types of capability for suicide (dispositional, acquired, and practical), and it's helpful to explore how each relates to you. You can use this information to create more physical safety in your life.

- Creating emotional safety is also a key factor in effectively coping with suicidal thoughts. You can identify people you trust and communicate what you need. It's helpful when you can lean on others for support as you talk openly about your suicidal thoughts.

Reflection

What thoughts, ideas, and feelings did you have while reading and working through this chapter? Were there certain parts you didn't relate to? What parts did you relate to most? What did you learn?

CHAPTER 11

Plan for the Future

Congratulations! You made it to the last chapter of this workbook. I hope you are incredibly proud of yourself for working through these exercises. Your life and well-being are important, and I'm glad that you're making your mental health a priority. When you're struggling with suicidal thoughts, it is especially hard to find the energy to learn new coping strategies. You stuck with it and worked toward making real change. In this chapter, we'll revisit what you learned, reflect on the changes you have noticed, and make a plan to keep prioritizing your mental health.

Many people who experience suicidal thoughts have them return at other points in their lives. For some people, suicidal thoughts reemerge when their mental health worsens or if stressful events occur. For other people, suicidal thoughts pop into their minds even when they're not in a particularly emotionally painful state. I want you to be aware of this, so you don't think the return of suicidal thoughts means you are doing anything wrong or that you're alone in your experiences. Completing this workbook is not something that makes suicidal thoughts completely go away for everyone. Instead, I hope you will keep this as a resource that you can return to whenever you need it. You now have the tools to cope with suicidal thoughts if they return. The strategies in this book are skills that will stay sharpest if you continue to practice them regularly. I hope they will provide you with a sense of peace and confidence in your ability to work through life's hardships.

The Tools You Have Learned

In chapter 1, you read an overview on how to use the book and an introduction to CBT. You gained insight into the ways your thoughts, emotions, and behaviors are linked and influence each other. I hope you felt empowered to find new, effective ways to cope with suicidal thoughts. Let's take a moment to reflect on chapter 1. Which thinking patterns are you most prone to? List them below so you remember to look out for them in the future. Thanks to all your hard work, you know how to address them when they do happen (through the reframing strategies in chapter 5).

- _____

- _____

- _____

- _____
- _____
- _____

Next, chapter 2 helped you understand that you are not alone in your suicidal thoughts. You explored societal factors that influence your well-being and deepened your self-understanding. You learned that you are not to blame for your struggles.

After putting your experiences into context, we explored the causes of your suicidal thoughts and the pain underneath them in chapter 3. Some people have the same causes underlying suicidal thoughts throughout their lives, while others have causes that change over time. Chapter 3 is there for you to revisit any time you need to clarify the current sources of your pain.

You worked hard in chapter 4 to develop a plan for coping with crises. That is your toolkit for making it through the most intensely suicidal times. Please keep that crisis plan accessible wherever you are so that you will have a plan ready in your most painful moments. As discussed throughout the workbook, suicide prevention isn't just about keeping you alive, it's about making your life hurt less so that you want to be alive. That is why the book also focuses on how to create a life you want to live.

In chapter 5, you learned problem solving and CBT strategies for reducing emotional pain. In chapter 6, you learned how to do this while being friendly, loving, and accepting toward yourself. Self-compassion and acceptance are not easy for most of us. You may have had traumatic and painful experiences in which people told you that you were undeserving. Those experiences shape people and make it hard to shake self-criticism. Try to be patient with yourself as you try this new way of relating to yourself. Repeated practice will make it easier over time. If there is any skill in this workbook I'd ask that you practice every week or even every day, it's taking a moment to act in a friendly manner toward yourself. It doesn't have to be perfect. You don't have to go from feeling down to feeling 100 percent confident. The goal is to learn how to encourage yourself as you face life's struggles. You'll learn that life feels better when you're not layering harsh self-criticism on top of all your other stresses.

Suicide can start seeming like an escape to people who have lost hope in ever having a good life. Chapter 7 taught you the HOPE acronym (seek Help, find Optimism, change Perspective, attend to Emotions) so that you can use those skills whenever you need to build more hope in your life. Let's pause right here and reflect on how to apply those skills.

How I can use these skills to continuing building hope when life seems too hard:

_____

_____

What makes me hopeful for the future:

_____

_____

    Another core message of the workbook is this: humans need each other to thrive. In chapters 8 and 9, you learned how to strengthen the connections in your life through relationships, roles, and projects. In chapter 10, you learned how to do all of this while creating an environment with the physical and emotional safety you need. As you read through this concluding chapter, which ties the book's themes together, I hope a sense of accomplishment is growing within you. Look at all the work you have done to create a better life for yourself! That is truly impressive.

Changes You Have Made

I want to thank you for putting your faith and effort into this journey. You have learned how to strengthen your relationships, cultivate joy and self-compassion, problem solve, and practice many other tools for addressing the hardships in your life. I truly hope your life is richer for this experience. Let's take some time to reflect on the effects of those changes on your life with the exercise below (Jakobsons et al., 2007).

Change Check-In

Suicidal thoughts

How frequent are your suicidal thoughts as compared to when you first started reading the book? Circle your answer below:

More   Less   Same

How intense are your suicidal thoughts as compared to when you started the book? For example, do they tend to last as long? Are they less distressing than they used to be? Do they tend to be more passive and less active? Explore these questions and then write responses to them in the space below.

_____

_____

_____

_____

How long ago did you start using this book? At what point did you start noticing changes? Were there certain exercises or chapters that made the most impact? Reflect on these questions and write your thoughts in the space below.

_____

_____

Do you feel more equipped to cope with your suicidal thoughts after the process of going through this workbook? If yes, how so?

_____

_____

Changes in functioning

Have you noticed changes in how you're doing in different parts of your life since the beginning of this book? Circle the level of functioning that applies to each below:

School	n/a	better	the same	worse
Work	n/a	better	the same	worse
Family	n/a	better	the same	worse
Friendships	n/a	better	the same	worse
Romantic relationships	n/a	better	the same	worse
Physical health	n/a	better	the same	worse
Other areas	n/a	better	the same	worse

Why you feel different

If you have experienced changes, what do you think caused them? What have you done differently to make your life better? If your suicidal thoughts and functioning have worsened, why is that? Did you have stressful events happen in your life during the course of the workbook that increased your suffering? Did you have a hard time applying and practicing the skills? If so, I recommend reaching out to a therapist to help you with fitting the skills into your life. It can be hard to do on your own! Reflect on these questions in the space below.

_____

_____

_____

_____

_____

Using new skills

Are there times that stand out where you used your skills, and they were especially helpful? Have you found yourself in situations that used to be really challenging and discovered that you can now navigate them with your skills? Take some time to write about that below.

_____

_____

_____

_____

Confidence and pride

When people start therapy or a self-help workbook, it's common to feel doubtful that it will be useful for you. That is natural when you have tried other approaches that haven't worked. Is that how you felt before reading this book? If so, has that changed? Do you feel a greater sense of confidence in your ability to cope with suicidal thoughts now? Do you feel pride in what you have learned? Explore your thoughts and feelings in the space below.

_____

_____

_____

_____

Ripple effects

Have you found that any of the tools have helped in areas of your life outside of suicidal thoughts? For example, has self-compassion helped you cope with anxiety? Have the strategies for coping with hard emotions worked when you have felt irritable or angry too? Write about any ways that these skills have applied in other parts of your life.

_____

_____

Your Mental Health Is a Priority

If you took perfect care of your physical health for a year and then stopped eating nutritious foods for a few months, your body would suffer. If you regularly jogged for two years and then stopped for a few months, your jogging performance would decline. With physical health, we know that check-ups, activity, and eating well are necessary for maintaining gains. Your mental health is no different. If you don't prioritize your well-being and stop practicing your skills, your mental health will suffer. Mental health is much like physical health; it is something that needs tending to almost every day. This is especially true during highly stressful times. In order to prevent that from happening, let's make a plan for mental health maintenance.

My Mental Health Plan

As with all activities in this book, know that this plan is flexible and can be changed as life circumstances change. You may also need to tweak aspects of it as you learn what is most helpful to you. With mental health, there is usually a process of trying different things until you strike the right balance. As you write out your mental health maintenance plan, it's important to pick realistic goals that you can achieve. Small daily actions can help you stay on track. (A copy of this worksheet is available on the New Harbinger website for downloading and printing: http://www.newharbinger.com/47025.)

- What can you do on a daily basis to take care of your mental health? Will you aim for a certain number of hours of sleep each night? Are there eating habits that help you feel most healthy? How about tending to your relationships?

_____

_____

_____

_____

- What can you do on a weekly basis to take care of your mental health? Do you find that certain activities help you maintain a sense of meaning and positive mood (e.g., planning fun events, spending time with friends, meeting with a therapist)?

  _____

  _____

  _____

  _____

- What are some of your long-term goals (e.g., monthly or yearly)? Are there certain growth areas or milestones you want to strive for?

  _____

  _____

  _____

  _____

- What kind of obstacles and setbacks could get in the way of your mental health maintenance plan?

  _____

  _____

  _____

  _____

- How can you work around those obstacles and setbacks when they happen? Are there people you can ask for help? Can you adjust your goals so that they are more fitting for your current situation? Brainstorm possible solutions for each obstacle.

  _____

  _____

  _____

  _____

- Remember to check in with yourself, your feelings, and your suicidal thoughts regularly so that you can address your needs by revisiting certain chapters in the book (e.g., if you're feeling especially self-critical, you can open up chapter 6 as a reminder of exercises for coping with that).

Closing Thoughts

From the bottom of my heart, I want to thank you for investing in your mental health. I dug deep into the research literature and my experiences as a therapist to share everything I have learned about helping people with suicidal thoughts. I hope that all the effort and time you have invested in this workbook has changed your life for the better. I want you to feel empowered by all of the tools and skills you've gained through your hard work. I'm grateful that you gave it a chance. I'm wishing you a future filled with joy, meaning, and hope!

Summary of Key Points

- Mental health requires continual attention and care.

- You have skills and tools to get through tough times. You will make mistakes. We all do. It's important to be loving and compassionate toward yourself when you do and then find a way to get back on track.

- Creating a mental health plan makes it easier to stick with maintaining your gains and improving the future.

Reflection

What thoughts, ideas, and feelings did you have while reading and working through this chapter? Were there certain parts you didn't relate to? What parts did you relate to most? What did you learn?

A Note to Concerned Friends and Family Members

If you are reading this book out of concern for someone you care about, please know that your support can make a difference in the life of the person who is suffering. One of the heartbreaking aspects of suicide is that deeply loved people feel utterly alone and hopeless. In addition, they may lack the energy to reach out to others, or they may feel unworthy of help. I hope that this workbook helps you better understand the person you are concerned about.

In this appendix, I answer the most common questions I have been asked over the years. My responses are shaped from listening to people who have firsthand experiences with suicidal crises, from my clinical experiences with patients, and from years of conducting research on suicidal thoughts and behavior. There are always individual circumstances to consider, because suicidal thoughts affect all kinds of people in all kinds of different situations. My guiding principle is to be as ethical, humane, and effective as possible. That means treating people with dignity, respecting their autonomy, and prioritizing their input about what they find most helpful.

It's important to remember that people want to kill themselves because their lives hurt. Safety is important—lifesaving even—and chapter 10 focuses on that, but we must also think of the emotional and mental health impact of our actions beyond managing emergency moments. Our own fear, distress, and urgency can interfere with our ability to step back and figure out what would be most helpful to the person both during a crisis and in the long term. That is understandable and something you can work through even though it means tolerating some discomfort during the process. People with suicidal thoughts often simply want to be heard; they want to express themselves without feeling judged or misunderstood. Remember that many people experience suicidal thoughts and that the majority do not attempt suicide. The thoughts still cause distress even if the person having them doesn't intend to act on them, and thus they still warrant support and care. You can do a lot for a person simply by listening, learning about their experiences, and asking how you can best support them. With those points in mind, below are my answers to common questions.

What Warning Signs Should I Look For?

Research suggests that we need more scientific work to improve our understanding of the most relevant risk factors and warning signs for suicide (Franklin et al., 2017). Part of the challenge is that other people cannot always see signs that someone is struggling from the outside. With that context, here are some possible warning signs to look for (American Association of Suicidology, 2020; Chu et al., 2015):

- talking about wanting to kill themselves

- looking for ways to kill themselves (e.g., trying to get a gun or other suicide methods)

- talking or writing about death more than usual

- increased use of alcohol or other substances

- expressing that they have no purpose or reason for living

- high levels of agitation

- saying that they feel trapped or hopeless

- increased sleep disturbances (e.g., nightmares, insomnia)

- significant weight loss without intention to lose weight

- withdrawing from others

- increase in reckless behavior

- extreme mood changes

- giving away important belongings (including pets)

- neglecting basic self-care and hygiene

What Should I Do If I See Warning Signs?

Open the discussion by asking them how they're feeling and be direct about your concerns that they're suicidal. Research shows that this can be helpful and will not plant the idea in their head (Blades et al., 2018). Then listen nonjudgmentally to their response. It's painful to hear someone say they're thinking of killing themselves or that they want to die, yet it's important to try to continue to listen without judgment. Express support and compassion. You can do this with words, but often people express empathy through nonverbal facial expressions and gestures too. It can be as simple as reminding them that you love them, asking questions to show that you genuinely want to understand, and acknowledging their pain as a valid experience. Once you have given them an opportunity to describe how they're feeling, ask what they think would be helpful before jumping in with advice.

Below I'll share some suggestions that are based on what people with suicidal thoughts and behaviors have told me feels good (and bad) to them.

Typically unhelpful:

- "You have so many wonderful things in your life. You should be more grateful."

- "Other people have it much harder than you. What do you have to be so upset about?"

- "You need to just focus on the positive and stop dwelling on negative thoughts."

- "Whenever I feel down, I just go work out [or pray, go to yoga, say affirmations, look at the bright side, meditate, eat healthy, etc.], and I feel better. You should do that."

- "You can't let these things get to you. You're overthinking things."

- "You're just doing this for attention. It would be selfish for you to do that to your family."

- "We need to call 911 or take you to the hospital!" [If this is said without first having a discussion with the person about why they're feeling the way they do and whether they are currently physically safe.]

- "You'll be fine."

Typically helpful:

- "It sounds like you're in a lot of pain. What's hurting right now?"

- "I love you and care about you. I want to understand what you're going through."

- "You're not alone in this. Other people struggle with this too."

- "It's not your fault that you feel this way. There's no reason to feel ashamed."

- "I'm really glad that you're opening up to me about this. That takes courage."

- "What can I do to support you?"

- "It means a lot that you're sharing your feelings with me. I would like to hear more if you're comfortable telling me."

- "If I were in your position, I think I would feel that way too. I'm not sure how I would cope with it."

After opening the conversation, listening, and expressing support, find ways to reassure them realistically and work together to form an action plan. For example:

- "You're not alone in this. I'll do the best I can to help you through this."

- "You have been through a lot before. It might be hard for you to see this right now, but I believe you can get through this. I'll help in any way I can."

- "Have you tried things in the past that helped you? Are there some we can try again?"

- "I'm worried about losing you. You mean so much to me. How can we make sure you're safe?" [Like reduce access to firearms, medications, and other methods for suicide, see chapter 10.]

- "What's one small step that would help you feel better?" [Like spend time together, create a hope kit (see chapter 7), pick an enjoyable hobby, go for a walk, call a friend, make plans to seek treatment.]

- "I'm glad you're talking to me now, but I also want to make sure that you have people you can turn to if I'm unavailable or you just want to reach out to someone else. Are there other people you could reach out to? If you don't have friends you feel comfortable talking with, there's a hotline number you can call too: 1-800-273-TALK."

- "Seeking professional help may seem like a lot right now, but I think it's worth trying. Can I help you connect with those services?"

- "If you're nervous about starting therapy, I can go with you. Just let me know how I can support you through the process."

What About Involuntary Hospitalization?

Some people ask, "The person I care about agreed to go to a therapist but is worried about involuntary hospitalization. How do mental health professionals make decisions about this?" Laws vary by location and the decision process depends on the particular mental health professional, patient, and situation. The typical criterion for involuntary hospitalization is that the person must be at immediate risk for suicide or hurting others. The mental health professionals whom I have interacted with over the years tend to be eager to find alternatives to involuntary hospitalization, unless the person is talking about specific plans to kill themselves within the next few days and cannot find a way to stop themselves. This is not always the case, so it's worth knowing that there is a chance of involuntary hospitalization. In my experience, however, it has been a small risk, because most mental health professionals I have encountered seek to respectfully and collaboratively create a safety plan with patients.

It's important to know that your loved one has the right to ask about these concerns and make an informed choice before meeting with a mental health professional. You can help them take steps beforehand to find out information about the particular mental health professional's approach. You can call and ask about their decision making about involuntary hospitalization and their expertise and experience working with patients with suicidal thoughts. Hopefully, you'll find that the therapist is transparent in responding to these questions. If not, you may consider seeking services with someone who can directly answer your questions.

Supporting My Loved One Is Affecting My Own Mental Health

Your mental health matters too. If you need to set some boundaries with your availability to help the person, that is okay. Take a step back and think about how you need to make more space for your own mental health. You may find it helpful to meet with your own therapist to learn how to balance supporting your loved one while tending to your needs as well. One possible way to approach this would be to say something to your friend or family member like, "I see that you're in a lot of pain, and I really feel for you. I can support you in certain ways right now, but I'm struggling to figure out how to take care of my mental health too. Can we think about some other people you might be able to rely on too? Let's think about friends, relatives, peer support, a therapist, or hotlines you can contact if I'm not available at the time. I care about you, and it's important to me that you find the support that you need when I can't provide as much as I would like." You can alter this to what fits you best, but the goal is to show that you are prioritizing mental health in your own life and want them to as well. You can show that you care while making sure that you are okay too.

I Lost Someone to Suicide. How Can I Cope with My Loss?

I am so sorry for your loss. The death of a loved one to suicide can be especially difficult because you know that the person was suffering. Sometimes, people blame themselves for not knowing something was wrong or for not doing more to prevent suicide. This appendix focuses on how we can each do our part to try to connect with our loved ones and help if they're having suicidal thoughts. However, we can't always know how much others are struggling. Even if we do know, we can't always stop them from taking their lives. That is a tragic part of suicide, but it's important that you know that and do not blame yourself. Ultimately, there are limitations to what any of us can do, even if we do all that is within our power. Please consider seeking therapy or a bereavement group specifically for people who have lost someone to suicide. In my experience, people find that they feel more understood and comforted when they talk to people who have gone through the same kind of heartbreak. Appendix B includes the American Association of Suicidology website, which has information specifically for people who have lost loved ones to suicide.

How Can I Learn More About Suicide Prevention?

You will find additional resources in appendix B.

Additional Resources

Books

Bryan, C., and M. D. Rudd. 2018. *Brief Cognitive-Behavioral Therapy for Suicide Prevention*. New York: The Guilford Press.

Burns, D. 1980. *Feeling Good: The New Mood Therapy*. New York: HarperCollins.

Freedenthal, S. 2018. *Helping the Suicidal Person*. New York: Routledge.

Gratz, K., and A. Chapman. 2009. *Freedom from Self-Harm: Overcoming Self-Injury with Skills from DBT and Other Treatments*. Oakland: New Harbinger.

Hershfield, J. 2018. *Overcoming Harm OCD: Mindfulness and CBT Tools for Coping with Unwanted Violent Thoughts*. Oakland: New Harbinger.

Jobes, D. 2016. *Managing Suicidal Risk: A Collaborative Approach*. 2nd ed. New York: The Guilford Press.

Joiner, T. 2005. *Why People Die by Suicide*. Cambridge: Harvard University Press.

Joiner, T., K. Van Orden, T. Witte, and M. D. Rudd. *The Interpersonal Theory of Suicide: Guidance for Working with Suicidal Clients*. Washington, DC: American Psychological Association.

Linehan, M. 1993. *Cognitive-Behavioral Treatment of Borderline Personality Disorder*. New York: The Guilford Press.

Linehan, M. 2015. *DBT Skills Training Manual*. 2nd ed. New York: The Guilford Press.

Minden, J. 2020. *Show Your Anxiety Who's Boss*. Oakland: New Harbinger.

Silberman, S. 2008. *The Insomnia Workbook*. Oakland: New Harbinger.

Singh, A. 2018. *The Queer & Transgender Resilience Workbook*. Oakland: New Harbinger.

Walker, R. 2020. *The Unapologetic Guide to Black Mental Health*. Oakland: New Harbinger.

Websites

American Association of Suicidology: https://suicidology.org

American Foundation for Suicide Prevention: https://afsp.org

Crisis Text Line: https://www.crisistextline.org

International Association for Suicide Prevention: https://www.iasp.info

International Society for the Study of Self-Injury: https://itriples.org

Live Through This: https://livethroughthis.org

Mental Health Art by Alyse Ruriani: https://alyseruriani.com

National Suicide Prevention Lifeline: https://suicidepreventionlifeline.org

The Psych Show with Dr. Ali Mattu: https://www.youtube.com/c/thepsychshow

Trans Lifeline: https://translifeline.org

The Trevor Project: https://www.thetrevorproject.org

Acknowledgments

I'm grateful to everyone who supported me, provided feedback, and shaped my thinking about suicidality. It is impossible to name everyone and stick to my word limit, but I want to especially thank:

- Keith, Lyla, Graham, and Maddy for encouragement, love, and time to write.

- Mom, Dad, Annie, and Linda—for being a family that discusses mental health openly and without stigma.

- My graduate school mentor, Thomas Joiner, for setting the bar high, leading by example, and believing in me.

- All of my past, present, and future patients for sharing their lives in our work together.

- My former NDSU students, especially the ones who I was fortunate to mentor and conduct suicide research with: Betsy Carter, Darren Carter, Valerie Douglas, Mun Yee Kwan, and Allison Minnich.

- My brilliant suicide prevention colleagues and friends: Ted Bender, Jill Holm-Denoma, April Smith, Kim Van Orden, and Tracy Witte.

- People who have shared their wisdom and mentored me at critical points in my education and career: Sandy Kerr, Tricia Myers, Marisol Perez, and Steve Wonderlich.

- Kelly Kismet McIntyre for supporting my writing and providing valuable feedback on an early draft of this workbook.

- Alyse Ruriani, the exceptional graphic designer and art therapist who created two beautiful illustrations for the workbook.

- David Klonsky, who answered my questions about the three-step theory and whose scientific contributions strongly influenced this workbook.

- Dese'Rae L. Stage, whose Live Through This project influenced this book by amplifying the voices and lived experiences of suicide attempt survivors for the public.

- Leigh Stein, whose Sunday newsletter about writing and the book publishing industry provided me with many useful tips and ideas.

- Everyone at New Harbinger who made this book possible and improved it along the way, particularly Ryan Buresh, Caleb Beckwith, and Jennifer Eastman.

- The supportive and funny friends who checked in with me during the time I wrote this workbook, especially Joel Minden, Leonardo Bobadilla, Yessenia Castro, Wendy Gordon, and Rob Gordon.

- My loving, fun relatives: Bill, Ceil, Ken, Madeline, John, Cora, Ollie, Ben, Jim, Jean, Lissa, Carly, Joe, Mary, Mark, Kayleigh, Maren, Theresa, Michelle, Aric, Jennifer, Amanda, Louise, Frank, Andy, Erin, Ellie, Bradley, Claire, Todd, Mary, Nina, Maggie, and Peggy.

- My beloved grandmother, Madge Marten, who knew all of the lessons in this workbook intuitively.

References

Abramson, L., G. Metalsky, and L. Alloy. 1989. "Hopelessness depression: A theory-based subtype of depression." *Psychological Review* 96: 358–372.

American Association of Suicidology. 2020. *Warning Signs.* https://suicidology.org/resources/warning-signs. Retrieved September 6, 2020.

Anestis, M. 2018. *Guns and Suicide: An American Epidemic.* New York: Oxford University Press.

Anestis, M., and C. Houtsma. 2017. "The association between gun ownership and statewide overall suicide rates." *Suicide and Life-Threatening Behavior* 48: 204–217.

Ashrafioun, L., T. Bishop, K. Conner, and W. Pigeon. 2017. "Frequency of description opioid misuse and suicidal ideation, planning, and attempts." *Journal of Psychiatric Research* 92: 1–7.

Beck, A. 1979. *Cognitive Therapy and the Emotional Disorders.* New York: Plume.

Beck, A. 1993. "Cognitive therapy: Past, present, and future." *Journal of Consulting and Clinical Psychology* 61: 194–198.

Bentley, K., M. Nock, and D. Barlow. 2014. "The four function model of nonsuicidal self-injury: Key directions for future research." *Clinical Psychological Science* 5: 638–656.

Blades, C., W. Stritzke, A. Page, and J. Brown. 2018. "The benefits and risks of asking research participants about suicide: A meta-analysis of the impact of exposure to suicide-related content." *Clinical Psychology Review* 64: 1–12.

Bluth, K., and K. Neff. 2018. "New frontiers in understanding the benefits of self-compassion." *Self and Identity* 6: 605–608.

Boness, C., R. Hershenberg, J. Kaye, M.A. Mackintosh, D. Grasso, A. Noser, and S. Raffa. 2020. "An evaluation of Cognitive Behavioral Therapy for Insomnia: A systematic review and application of Tolin's criteria for empirically supported treatments. *Clinical Psychology: Science and Practice.* Early view: e12348.

Bridge, J., L. Horowitz, C. Fontanella, A. Sheftall, J. Greenhouse, K. Kelleher, and J. Campo. 2018. "Age-related racial disparity in suicide rates among US youths from 2001 through 2015." *JAMA Pediatrics* 172(7): 697–699.

Britton, P., H. Patrick, A. Wenzel, and G. Williams. 2011. "Integrating motivational interviewing and self-determination theory with cognitive-behavioral therapy to prevent suicide." *Cognitive Behavioral Practice* 18: 16–27.

Bryan, C., A. Bryan, D. Rozek, and F. Keifker. 2019. "Meaning in life drives reductions in suicide risk among acutely suicidal soldiers receiving a crisis response plan." *Journal of Social and Clinical Psychology* 38: 774–787.

Bryan, C., and M. D. Rudd. 2018. *Brief Cognitive-Behavioral Therapy for Suicide Prevention.* New York: Guilford Press.

Burns, D. 1980. *Feeling Good: The New Mood Therapy.* New York: HarperCollins.

Bush, N., S. Dobscha, R. Crumptom, L. Denneson, J. Hoffman, A. Crain, R. Cromer, and J. Kinn. 2014. "A virtual hope box smartphone app as an accessory to therapy: A proof-of-concept in a clinical sample of veterans." *Suicide and Life-Threatening Behavior* 45: 1–9.

Cerel, J., M. Brown, M. Maple, M. Singleton, J. Van de Venne, M. Moore, and C. Flaherty. 2018. "How many people are exposed to suicide? Not six." *Suicide and Life-Threatening Behavior* 49: 529–534.

Chesney, E., G. Goodwin, and S. Fazel. (2014). "Risks of all-cause and suicide mortality in mental disorders: A meta-review." *World Psychiatry* 13: 153–160.

Chu, C., J. Buchman-Schmitt, I. Stanley, M. Hom, R. Tucker, C. Hagan, M. Rogers, M. Podlogar, B. Chiurliza, F. Ringer et al. 2017. "The interpersonal theory of suicide: A systematic review and meta-analysis of a decade of cross-national research." *Psychological Bulletin* 143: 1313–1345.

Chu, C., K. Klein, J. Buchman-Schmitt, M. Hom, C. Hagan, and T. Joiner. 2015. "Routinized assessment of suicide risk in clinical practice: An empirically informed update." *Journal of Clinical Psychology* 71: 1186–1200.

Cuijpers, P., C. Gentili, R. Banos, J. Garcia-Campayo, C. Botella, and I. Cristea. 2016. "Relative effects of cognitive and behavioral therapies on generalized anxiety disorder, social anxiety disorder, and panic disorder: A meta-analysis." *Journal of Anxiety Disorders* 43: 78–89.

Denneson, L, D. Smolénski, B. Bauer, S. Dobscha, and N. Bush. 2019. "The mediating role of coping self-efficacy in hope box use and suicidal ideation severity." *Archives of Suicide Research* 223: 234–246.

Dimidjian, S., S. Hollon, K. Dobson, K. Schmaling, R. Kohlenberg, M. Addis, R. Getallop, J. McGlinchey, D. Markley, J. Gollan et al. 2006. "Randomized trial of behavioral activation, cognitive therapy, and antidepressant medication in the acute treatment of adults with major depression." *Journal of Consulting and Clinical Psychology* 74: 658–670.

Drapeau, C., and J. McIntosh. 2020. *U.S.A. Suicide 2018: Official Final Data.* Washington, D.C.: American Association of Suicidology, https://suicidology.org/wp-content/uploads/2020/02/2018datapgsv2_Final.pdf.

Ellis, A. 2016. *How to Control Your Anxiety Before It Controls You.* New York: Citadel Press.

Frankl, V. 1955, 2006. *Man's Search for Meaning.* Boston: Beacon Press.

Franklin, J., J. Ribeiro, K. Fox, K. Bentley, E. Kleiman, X. Huang, K. Musacchio, A., Jaroszewski, B. Chang, and M. Nock. 2017. "Risk factors for suicidal thoughts and behaviors: A meta-analysis of 50 years of research." *Psychological Bulletin* 143: 187–232.

Gratz, K., and A. Chapman. 2009. *Freedom from Self-Harm: Overcoming Self-Injury with Skills from DBT and Other Treatments*. Oakland: New Harbinger.

Hames, J., J. Ribeiro, A. Smith, and T. Joiner. 2012. "An urge to jump affirms the urge to live: An empirical examination of the high place phenomenon." *Journal of Affective Disorders* 136: 1114–1120.

Han, B., P. Kott, A. Hughes, R. McKeon, C. Blanco, and W. Compton. 2016. "Estimating the rates of deaths by suicide among adults who attempt suicide in the United States." *Journal of Psychiatric Research* 77: 125–133.

Hanh, T. N. 1976. *The Miracle of Mindfulness: An Introduction to the Practice of Meditation*. Boston: Beacon Press.

Hershfield, J. 2018. *Overcoming Harm OCD: Mindfulness and CBT Tools for Coping with Unwanted Violent Thoughts*. Oakland: New Harbinger.

Holt-Lunstad, J., T. Smith, M. Baker, T. Harris, and D. Stephenson. 2015. "Loneliness and social isolation as risk factors for mortality: A meta-analytic review." *Perspectives on Psychological Science* 10: 227–237.

Hottes, T. S., L. Bogaert, A. Rhodes, D. Brennan, and D. Gesink. 2016. "Lifetime prevalence of suicide attempts among sexual minority adults by study sampling strategies: A systematic review and meta-analysis." *American Journal of Public Health* 106: e1–e12.

International Society for the Study of Self-Injury. 2019. *Who engages in self-injury?* https://itriples.org /about-self-injury/who-engages-in-self-injury. Retrieved December 22, 2019.

Jakobsons, L., J. Brown, K. Gordon, and T. Joiner. 2007. "When are clients ready to terminate?" *Cognitive and Behavioral Practice* 14: 218–230.

Joiner, T. 2005. *Why People Die by Suicide*. Cambridge: Harvard University Press.

Klonsky, E. D. 2007. "The functions of deliberate self-injury: A review of the evidence." *Clinical Psychology Review* 27: 226–239.

Klonsky, E. D., and A. May. 2015. "The Three-Step Theory (3ST): A new theory of suicide rooted in the 'Ideation-to-Action' framework." *International Journal of Cognitive Therapy* 8: 114–129.

Klonsky, E. D., A. May, and C. Glenn. 2013. "The relationship between nonsuicidal self-injury and attempted suicide: Converging evidence from four samples." *Journal of Abnormal Psychology* 122: 231–237.

Klonsky, E. D., A. May, and B. Saffer. 2016. "Suicide, suicide attempts, and suicidal ideation." *Annual Review of Clinical Psychology* 12: 307–30.

Krakow, B., and A. Zadra. 2010. "Clinical management of chronic nightmares: Imagery Rehearsal Therapy." *Behavioral Sleep Medicine* 4: 45–70.

Li, Z., A. Page., G. Martin, and R. Taylor. 2011. "Attributable risk of psychiatric and socioeconomic factors for suicide from individual-level, population-based studies: A systematic review." *Social Science & Medicine* 4: 608–616.

Lindsey, M., A. Sheftall, Y. Xio, and S. Joe. (2019). "Trends of suicidal behaviors among high school students in the United States: 1991–2017." *Pediatrics* 144(5): e20191187.

Linehan, M. 1993. *Cognitive-Behavioral Treatment of Borderline Personality Disorder.* New York: Guilford Press.

Linehan, M. 2020. *Building a Life Worth Living: A Memoir.* New York: Random House.

Liu, R., E. Kleiman, B. Nestor, and S. Creek. 2015. "The hopelessness theory of depression: A quarter century in review." *Clinical Psychology.* 22: 345–365.

Liu, R., S. Steele, J. Hamilton, D. Quyen, K. Furbish, T. Burke, A. Martinez, and N. Gerlus. 2020. "Sleep and suicide: A systematic review and meta-analysis of longitudinal studies." *Clinical Psychology Review* 81.

Marshall, E., L. Claes, W. Bouman, G. Whitcomb, and J. Arcelus. 2015. "Non-suicidal self-injury and suicidality in trans people: A systematic review of the literature." *International Review of Psychiatry* 28: 58–69.

Miller, W., and S. Rollnick. 2013. *Motivational Interviewing.* New York: Guilford Press.

Neff, K. 2003. "Self-compassion: An alternative conceptualization of a healthy attitude toward oneself." *Self and Identity* 2: 85–101.

Nock, M., I. Hwang, N. Sampson, and R. Kessler. 2009. "Mental disorders, comorbidity and suicidal behavior: Results from the National Comorbidity Survey Replication." *Molecular Psychiatry* 15: 868–876.

O'Connor, R. and M. Nock. 2014. "The psychology of suicidal behavior." *Lancet Psychiatry* 1: 73–85.

Oh, H., A. Stickley, A. Koyanagi, R. Yau, and J. DeVylder. (2019). "Discrimination and suicidality among racial and ethnic minorities in the United States." *Journal of Affective Disorders* 245: 517–523.

Opara, I., M. A. Assan, K. Pierre, J. Gunn, I. Metzger, J. Hamilton, and E. Arugu. 2020. "Suicide among Black children: An integrated model of the interpersonal-psychological theory of suicide and intersectionality theory for researchers and clinicians." *Journal of Black Studies* 51(6): 611–631.

Oquendo, M., and N. Volkow. 2018. "Suicide: A silent contributor to opioid-overdose deaths." *New England Journal of Medicine* 378: 1567–1569.

Owens, D., J. Horrocks, and A. House. 2002. "Fatal and non-fatal repetition of self-harm: A systematic review." *British Journal of Psychiatry* 18: 193–99.

Owens, S., and T. Eisenlohr-Moul. 2018. "Suicide risk and the menstrual cycle: A review of candidate RDoC mechanisms." *Current Psychiatry Reports* 20: 106.

Raifman, J., E. Moscoe, S. B. Austin, and M. McConnell. 2017. "Difference-in-differences analysis of the association between state same-sex marriage policies and adolescent suicide attempts." *JAMA Pediatrics* 171(4): 350–356.

Salway, T., M. Plöderl, J. Liu, and P. Gustafson. 2019. "Effects of multiple forms of information bias on estimated prevalence of suicide attempts according to sexual orientation: An application of a Bayesian misclassification correction method to data from a systematic review." *American Journal of Epidemiology* 188: 239–249.

Sand, B., K. Gordon, and K. Bresin. 2013. "The impact of specifying suicide as the cause of death in an obituary." *Crisis* 34: 63–66.

Selby, E., M. Anestis, and T. Joiner. 2007. "Daydreaming about death: Violent daydreaming as a form of emotion dysregulation in suicidality." *Behavior Modification* 6: 867–879.

Smith, A., T. Witte, and T. Joiner. 2010. "Reasons for cautious optimism? Two studies suggest reduced stigma against suicide." *Journal of Clinical Psychology* 66: 611–626.

Stanley, I., K. Rufino, M. Rogers, T. Ellis, and T. Joiner. 2016. "Acute Suicidal Affective Disturbance (ASAD): A confirmatory factor analysis with 1442 psychiatric inpatients." *Journal of Psychiatric Research* 80: 97–104.

Stickley, A., and A. Koyanagi. 2016. "Loneliness, common mental disorders and suicidal behavior: Findings from a general population survey." *Journal of Affective Disorders* 197: 81–87.

Stone, D., T. Simon, K. Fowler., S. Kegler, K. Yuan, K. Holland, A. Ivey-Stephenson, and A. Crosby. 2018. "Vital signs: Trends in the state suicide rates—United States, 1999–2016, and circumstances contributing to suicide—27 states, 2015." *MMWR Morbidity and Mortality Weekly Report* 67: 617–624.

Substance Abuse and Mental Health Services Administration. 2017. *Key Substance Use and Mental Health Indicators in the United States: Results from the 2016 National Survey on Drug Use and Health.* Retrieved from: www.samhsa.gov/data/sites/default/files/NSDUH-FFR1-2016/NSDUH-FFR1 -2016.pdf.

Swannell, S., G. Martin, A. Page, P. Hasking, and N. St. John. 2014. "Prevalence of nonsuicidal self-injury in nonclinical samples: A systematic review, meta-analysis, and meta-regression." *Suicide and Life-Threatening Behavior* 44: 273–303.

Tarrier, N., K. Taylor, and P. Gooding. 2008. "Cognitive-behavioral interventions to reduce suicide behavior: A systematic review and meta-analysis." *Behavior Modification* 32: 77–108.

Testa, R., M. Michaels, W. Bliss, M. Rogers, K. Balsam, and T. Joiner. 2017. "Suicidal ideation in transgender people: Gender minority stress and interpersonal theory factors." *Journal of Abnormal Psychology* 126: 125–136.

Van Orden, K., T. Witte, K. Cukrowicz, S. Braithwaite, E. Selby, and T. Joiner. 2010. "The interpersonal theory of suicide." *Psychological Review* 117: 575–600.

Weisskopf-Joelson, E. 1955. "Some comments on a Viennese school of psychiatry." *The Journal of Abnormal and Social Psychology* 51: 701–703.

Wenzel, A., G. Brown, and A. Beck. 2009. *Cognitive Therapy for Suicidal Patients: Scientific and Clinical Applications.* Washington, D.C.: American Psychological Association.

World Health Organization. 2019. *Suicide Fact Sheet.* Retrieved from: www.who.int/news-room /fact-sheets/detail/suicide. Retrieved December 14, 2019.

Yip, P., E. Caine, S. Yousuf, S. Change, W. Chien-Chang, and Y. Chen. 2012. "Means restriction for suicide prevention." *The Lancet* 379: 2393–2399.

Zalsman, G., K. Hawton, D. Wasserman, K. van Heeringen, E. Arensman, M. Sarchiapone, V. Carli, C. Hoschl, R. Barzilay, J. Balazs et al. 2016. "Suicide prevention strategies revisited: 10-year systematic review." *The Lancet: Psychiatry* 3: 646–659.

Kathryn Hope Gordon, PhD, is a licensed clinical psychologist who specializes in cognitive behavioral therapy (CBT). Prior to working as a therapist, Gordon was a professor for ten years. She is a mental health researcher who has published more than eighty scientific articles and book chapters on suicidal behavior, disordered eating, and related topics. Gordon cohosts the *Psychodrama* podcast, blogs for *Psychology Today*, and shares mental health information through her website: www.kathrynhgordon.com.

Foreword writer **Thomas Ellis Joiner, Jr., PhD**, is Bright-Burton professor of psychology, and director of the University Psychology Clinic at Florida State University. He has served as associate editor of the *Journal of Behavior Therapy*; and sits on ten editorial boards, including that of the *Journal of Consulting and Clinical Psychology*.

Real Change *Is* Possible

For more than forty-five years, New Harbinger has
published proven-effective self-help books and pioneering
workbooks to help readers of all ages and backgrounds
improve mental health and well-being, and achieve lasting
personal growth. In addition, our spirituality books
offer profound guidance for deepening awareness and
cultivating healing, self-discovery, and fulfillment.

Founded by psychologist Matthew McKay and Patrick
Fanning, New Harbinger is proud to be an independent,
employee-owned company. Our books reflect our
core values of integrity, innovation, commitment,
sustainability, compassion, and trust. Written by leaders
in the field and recommended by therapists worldwide,
New Harbinger books are practical, accessible, and
provide real tools for real change.

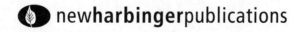 **newharbinger**publications

FROM OUR PUBLISHER—

As the publisher at New Harbinger and a clinical psychologist since 1978, I know that emotional problems are best helped with evidence-based therapies. These are the treatments derived from scientific research (randomized controlled trials) that show what works. Whether these treatments are delivered by trained clinicians or found in a self-help book, they are designed to provide you with proven strategies to overcome your problem.

Therapies that aren't evidence-based—whether offered by clinicians or in books—are much less likely to help. In fact, therapies that aren't guided by science may not help you at all. That's why this New Harbinger book is based on scientific evidence that the treatment can relieve emotional pain.

This is important: if this book isn't enough, and you need the help of a skilled therapist, use the following resources to find a clinician trained in the evidence-based protocols appropriate for your problem. And if you need more support—a community that understands what you're going through and can show you ways to cope—resources for that are provided below, as well.

Real help is available for the problems you have been struggling with. The skills you can learn from evidence-based therapies will change your life.

Matthew McKay, PhD
Publisher, New Harbinger Publications

If you need a therapist, the following organization can help you find a therapist trained in cognitive behavioral therapy (CBT).

The Association for Behavioral & Cognitive Therapies (ABCT) Find-a-Therapist service offers a list of therapists schooled in CBT techniques. Therapists listed are licensed professionals who have met the membership requirements of ABCT and who have chosen to appear in the directory.
Please visit www.abct.org and click on *Find a Therapist*.

National Suicide Prevention Lifeline
**Call 24 hours a day 1-800-273-TALK (8255)
or visit www.suicidepreventionlifeline.org**

MORE BOOKS from
NEW HARBINGER PUBLICATIONS

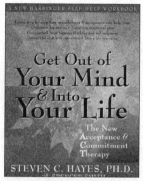
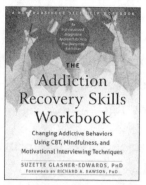
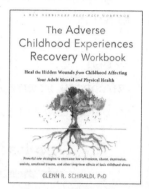
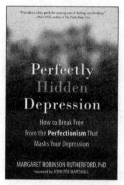
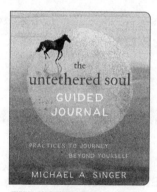
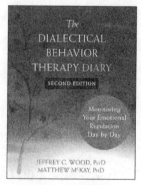

Register your **new harbinger** titles for additional benefits!

When you register your **new harbinger** title—purchased in any format, from any source—you get access to benefits like the following:

- Downloadable accessories like printable worksheets and extra content

- Instructional videos and audio files

- Information about updates, corrections, and new editions

Not every title has accessories, but we're adding new material all the time.

Access free accessories in 3 easy steps:

1. Sign in at NewHarbinger.com (or **register** to create an account).

2. Click on **register a book**. Search for your title and click the **register** button when it appears.

3. Click on the **book cover or title** to go to its details page. Click on **accessories** to view and access files.

That's all there is to it!

If you need help, visit:

NewHarbinger.com/accessories

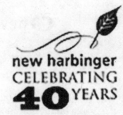

new harbinger
CELEBRATING
40 YEARS